Type 2 Diabetes

*Social and Scientific Origins,
Medical Complications and
Implications for Patients and Others*

ANDREW KAGAN, M.D., F.A.C.S.

*Forewords by Henry J. Heimlich, M.D.,
and Edward Asner*

McFarland & Company, Inc., Publishers
Jefferson, North Carolina, and London

LIBRARY OF CONGRESS CATALOGUING-IN-PUBLICATION DATA

Kagan, Andrew, 1941–
    Type 2 diabetes : social and scientific origins, medical
complications and implications for patients and others /
Andrew Kagan ; forewords by Henry J. Heimlich and
Edward Asner.
        p.   cm.
    Includes bibliographical references and index.

    ISBN 978-0-7864-4542-4
    softcover : 50# alkaline paper ∞

    1. Non-insulin-dependent diabetes.   I. Title.
    [DNLM: 1. Diabetes Mellitus, Type 2 — Case Reports.
    2. Diabetes Complications — Case Reports.   3. Quality of
    Life — Case Reports. WK 810K113t 2009]
    RC662.15.K34   2010
    616.4'624 — dc22   2009033387

British Library cataloguing data are available

Cover illustration: *Race and Ethnicity* by Andrew Kagan

Manufactured in the United States of America

McFarland & Company, Inc., Publishers
 Box 611, Jefferson, North Carolina 28640
  www.mcfarlandpub.com

For those who are,
those who were,
and those who will be

Give me health and a day, and I will make the pomp of emperors ridiculous.

— Ralph Waldo Emerson

ACKNOWLEDGMENTS

Thanks to the legions of diabetics who trusted me in body and spirit.

Thanks to my family for putting up with my absence for thirty-five years of solo surgical practice and their support in writing this book, and to Jeff Davis for his literary help.

Thanks to the fine physicians, nurses, and staff of the Hackensack University Hospital for the privilege of working with them and especially to Drs. Martin Blechman and Charlotte Sokol.

And special thanks to Arnold and Arlene Newman. Their constant encouragement is the impetus behind this book.

CONTENTS

FOREWORD

by Henry J. Heimlich, M.D.

It has become increasingly evident that an individual's genetic makeup is a major determinant of the course of his future medical history and a dominant factor in his longevity. This fact is particularly true in the case of type 2 diabetes. Now, in the twenty-first century, it is possible through scientific research to alter one's genetic profile, to check potential parents for hidden genetic defects in their unborn offspring and, potentially, to treat genetically induced diseases by employing gene therapy. This has already been accomplished in experimental animals and shows great promise in the treatment of genetically induced human illness. Until gene therapy becomes available, however, this book informs the reader what he or she can do to prevent type 2 diabetes or overcome the complications.

Type 2 diabetes afflicts close to 250 million people in the world today, 27 million in the United States alone. The worldwide incidence of type 2 diabetes is increasing in epidemic proportions. One of three children born today, at some stage in their lives, will become diabetic and develop disabling or fatal complications of the disease.

Type 2 diabetes is often underestimated in its potential to cause debilitating complications: heart disease, kidney failure, vascular disease, amputations, blindness and a host of additional physical impairments, all of which lead to premature demise. The object of Dr. Kagan's book is to educate and thereby empower the diabetic. The underlying premise is that, unlike many other disease suffers, diabetic patients must play a major role in order to alter the course of their disease. This is not possible without having a basic understanding of how diabetes affects each organ and why it causes early death. The educated diabetic is afforded the opportunity to minimize the complications and occasionally eliminate his disease.

Diabetes is not usually thought of as a surgical disease; however, almost every diabetic complication requires the input of a surgeon. To educate the reader, Dr. Kagan presents the facts in a unique fashion. He discusses specific cases, taken from his own 35-year surgical practice, which illustrate each type of complication. With each case presentation he incorporates an explanation of the cause and treatment, and when possible, of how to avoid complication.

It is Dr. Kagan's contention that diabetic patients must have a basic understanding of their disease, because ultimately it is the diabetic patients, by their own informed choices, who determine how to avoid the complications or at least minimize them.

Note well that the introduction in this book is no substitute for consulting your physician for medical advice and treatment Never disregard or delay seeking professional medical advice or treatment for something you have read about in this book.

Norman Vincent Peale declared that Dr. Heimlich has saved more lives than any other living person. The Heimlich Maneuver is known to save choking victims; it can save drowning victims by expelling water from the lungs and can stop or prevent asthma attacks. These and other discoveries are described in his forthcoming book, *Heimlich's Maneuvers*.

FOREWORD

by Edward Asner

Noting the rise in diabetes especially in the young, having a father, brother and friends who suffer with it and lastly enjoying the beauty of my six grandkids, it was imperative I have this book.

Dr. Kagan is a general/vascular surgeon with a 35 year niche practice in treating the complications of diabetes. He informs us that the various forms of diabetes have "emerged to be one of the most common and often mismanaged diseases on the planet." We have come to know that an increasingly unhealthy diet and sedentary lifestyle have contributed to cause the affliction in over 18,000,000 people in the United States where one third of its citizens are at risk for developing the disease. It is safe to say that this debilitating disease is developing in epidemic proportions and no particular sector of humanity is immune. Such an evolution means that few families will be untouched by diabetes mellitus.

This tragedy is exacerbated not only by the need to properly manage the disease, but deal effectively with the myriad complications that commonly plague the diabetic. Among the more serious of these are heart problems, blindness and vascular and nerve degeneration which commonly result in persistent ulcers and amputation.

One would think that with such a significant sector of the population suffering from this disease, and no shortage of books on the subject, there would hardly be a need for yet another. But this is assuredly not the case. Dr. Kagan's book is not a management guide for the diabetic patient. It is a highly readable account of case studies which inform us on not only the dramatic complications of this insidious disease, but also, more importantly, suggests how the patient, their families and their healthcare professionals can save life and limb by learning how to avoid and mitigate these complications. It is written by a leading surgeon in this field who has observed all the avoidable mistakes.

Diabetic?... Be enlightened!

Edward Asner is an award-winning television and film actor and a former president of the Screen Actors Guild. As a humanitarian he has lent his support to causes he believes in, and promoting the awareness of diabetes, with its grave complications, is one of them.

PREFACE

I am sure you've noticed that type 2 diabetes is getting a lot of attention these days, both in the form of ads for medications and glucose monitoring equipment as well as in newspaper articles, e-mails, magazines for diabetics, and requests for donations for diabetes research. Here in the United States we have an ever expanding subculture of type 2 diabetics. Hardly a family goes unaffected.

Booksellers' shelves, with good reason, are loaded with material to help type 2 diabetics navigate the course of their disease. This book, however, is not a reference manual or a treatment guide, these are stories, told through interesting case histories, which define the underlying biologic mechanisms that diabetics need to know in order to avoid the complications, and that prediabetics must be aware of in order to delay or avert the onset. The book aims to enlighten a vulnerable public so that others can avoid the environmental risks and stay off the list of 250 million people worldwide who already live with the disease.

This book has two parts; the first explains the environmental, biologic, and genetic origins of the disease, and provides an understandable account of the scientific and socioeconomic underpinning of the epidemic. The second part explores the diabetic's plight through surgical eyes, revealing the many causes and complications by using actual case histories, operating room encounters, and the life-altering experiences of several of my type 2 diabetic patients (all names have been changed). We surgeons have a unique perspective; we deal with the complications of insulin metabolism gone wrong, and we can not help but wonder: why did this happen, why is one out of five hospitalized patients diabetic, why is diabetes becoming the most common surgical disease on our planet?

The number of diabetics in the U.S., presently 27 million, will double within a generation in large part because the risk factors for developing the disease have become pervasive. The rapid increase has led the United States Centers for Disease Control to assume that, with regard to type 2 diabetes, there will be "no advances in prevention, no possibility of a cure, no increases in life expectancy, no increases in screening or changes in diagnostic criteria." A gloomy forecast indeed for those who are not enlightened.

Type 2 diabetes, unlike type 1, often begins as a silent condition. Unsuspecting patients may be lulled into complacency and blind to the machinations of their deranged metabolisms, which, if allowed to incubate, will produce grave physical complications — surgical complications. Once, it was believed that type 2 diabetes was limited to obese, sedentary people on fast food diets; today this is not the case. Today your socioeconomic status no longer protects you and being overweight is only one of many risk factors. Type 2 diabetes may be the result of various causes: a heavy genetic load, race, conditions surrounding your pregnancy (or your mother's pregnancy), a pre-existing disease, the medications you take for one malady or another, and most important — the diabetogenic effect of our industrialized world.

For thirty-five years as a vascular surgeon I have operated and taught medical students and surgical residents in one of the nation's largest hospitals, the Hackensack University Medical Center, primary teaching facility of the University of Medicine and Dentistry of New Jersey. In that time I have focused my work on treating the complications of diabetes (most of which are surgical). My work and my lectures for the Diabetes Federation of New Jersey have alerted me to the fears of experts in the fields of diabetes research and treatment. They are bracing for an overwhelming, worldwide health catastrophe. Nevertheless, it has been proven that those who understand the disease can side-step the risks and avoid or at least delay its arrival, and those already affected can minimize the complications.

INTRODUCTION

Ralph Waldo Emerson was quite familiar with illness and death when he put words to the timeless plea, used as the epigraph to this book: "Give me health and a day and I will make the pomp of emperors ridiculous."[1] No doubt, he was moved to write them by the loss, at age 8, of his father, and later of his first wife, Ellen Tucker, to tuberculosis, or consumption as it was called. She was nineteen. Soon after Emerson remarried, his first son, Waldo, succumbed to scarlet fever. Three of his four brothers lived brief, unhealthy lives and he himself was plagued by respiratory illness, probably bronchitis, until age thirty.

In Emerson's day, the natural environment was rife with uncontrollable health risks; back then, a long, healthy life was indeed a rare gift, as physicians had little but compassion to offer. In the 118 years since Emerson's death, scientific research and modern medicine have steadily evolved. In developed countries, many once-fatal childhood illnesses — polio, smallpox, tetanus, and tuberculosis (in the immunologically stable) to name a few — have been virtually eliminated. For those with chronic disease, like type 1 diabetes, modern medical know-how has made life sustainable, though not always comfortable. Life expectancy in America has increased from less than 50 years before the Civil War to near 80 today — a testament to our species, *Homo sapiens* (smart man).

While medical science has been busy conquering many of the 'natural' diseases, the industrialization of our food supply and transportation systems have evolved to sustain a growing world population. We call this progress, but progress, ironically, has its own unintended and unhealthy consequences. Through progress we have unwittingly converted our natural environment to an artificial one — and the by-product of an artificial environment is unnatural disease. Each year one and a quarter million of the world's people die in automobile accidents. Big-city asthma is rampant, industrial carcinogens cause deadly havoc, autism is rising, and the detrimental effects of obesity are tipping the balance of our healthcare system. These are only a handful of the harmful health by-products of our artificial environment.

Today's medical know-how, bio-technological breakthroughs, and pharmacological stop-gaps struggle to keep an entirely new set of environmental afflictions in check. One health hazard, it can be said, comes in under the radar, yet it commands the attention of every type of physician and affects 250 million people worldwide. Patients underestimate it as a serious disease (at least until its complications appear) and physicians, only now, recognize it as a healthcare catastrophe. Its pernicious role in premature heart disease, amputations, kidney failure, stroke and early death from a host of additional afflictions has become painfully apparent — it is type 2 diabetes, a disease deep-rooted in our industrial age.

Too often, life with type 2 diabetes is drug dependent and punctuated with surgeries — an existence quite evident to the world's quarter billion sufferers, and on one Sunday morning especially real to Annie Walker, as she lay on her back waiting while the nurse checked her chart. "We're ready," the nurse said, as she slipped the chart beneath Annie's pillow, unlocked the wheels and began to push. The gurney lurched forward. Annie gripped the steel side rails as it sailed past closed doors and down a narrow hallway. The glare of passing ceiling lights forced her eyes shut, but they quickly sprang open when the gurney swerved into the cold, antiseptic air of operating room 16. Jenny, the scrub nurse, relocked the wheels and lowered the side rails. Then she patted the white-sheeted operating table and beckoned her over. Dr. Leary, the anesthesiologist, leaned above her head, gently cupped her cheeks between gloved hands and tried, in a whisper, to comfort her. "You'll be fine Mrs. Walker; we'll take good care of you." She saw his eyes narrow and sensed a sympathetic smile beneath his mask. Jenny fetched a blanket from the warmer and wrapped it over her. It stopped the shivering, but failed to slow her heart or ease her thoughts. How could she, an educated woman, end up like this? Was she to blame? *No, of course not*, her conscience told her; *it was beyond her control*. She felt a burning in her arm. She tried to turn her head. It was too heavy. She opened her mouth to speak, but sleep, involuntary sleep, overtook her before any words escaped.

For thirty-five years I've practiced surgery in a very large, 1,000-bed, university-affiliated teaching-hospital — Annie Walker's hospital. Her case history, we shall see, is one of many that help explain why type 2 diabetes has become the most common disease of the twenty-first century. Our hospital sits on a hill overlooking New York City. It opened one hundred years ago — when surgery was still an art — and served a small, working-class community. When the suburban population began to swell, the hospital swallowed up a small neighborhood where single-family houses once stood. Now the fifth largest hospital in the United States, it continues to grow and take in the sick and injured from the most densely populated county in the most densely populated state in the nation, Bergen County, New Jersey. (Bergen County has the population of Alaska and Montana combined.)

When I began my surgical career in the early 1970s, modern pharmacological advances and expensive new medical technologies were beginning to transform the art of surgery into a technological business. In order to accommodate the health needs of a growing population and better serve those new technologies, the number of physicians on our hospital staff increased to well over 1,300. Now, in the early twenty-first century, the use of space-age diagnostic and therapeutic medical technology is the norm. There is still a place, though, for the often overlooked healing art of surgery.

The upside of advanced medical technology, pharmacology, and surgical know-how is a greater cure rate, the elimination of many diseases, and the prolongation of life. The downside is a gradual loss of the compassionate, one-on-one doctor-patient relationship. In our market-economy the seeker of medical care has become a healthcare consumer, and the physician, the surgeon in particular, has been converted from a devoted, science-based artisan to a shift-working, though still dedicated, bio-technologist. The bond between physician and patient is no longer physical; it's mechanical. The hands-on, meticulous physical exam has, for the most part, been replaced by the CAT scan, the MRI, the ultrasound, and the angiogram.

Type 1 diabetes mellitus, which was fatal in the 1920s, has, with the introduction of insulin, been transformed into a treatable disease with expected longterm survival. During the course of my surgical career, type 2 diabetes has become one of the most common, under-diagnosed, and mismanaged diseases on the planet. Today over 27 million Americans have type 2 diabetes and, according to the World Health Organization and the statistical forecast of the American Diabetes Association, within twenty-five to thirty years, half the adults in this country will live with this disease because it is a by-product of our way of life. Could Annie Walker have avoided it? Could you avoid an approaching tidal wave if you lived by the sea?

The basic biologic distinction between types 1 and 2 is this: type 1 diabetes stems from an unavoidable genetic flaw that alters one's metabolism. Type 2 arises from a metabolic defect, often environmentally induced but sometimes unwittingly self-imposed, that awakens a dormant genetic defect. In either case, the result is the same: a lack of or a malfunction of insulin, the hormone essential for normal organ function. The basic psychological distinction between type 1 and type 2 is this: type 1 diabetics know from the start that they have a serious disease; type 2s very often do not perceive the seriousness of their disease until a crisis arises.

Type 1 diabetes, I suspect, has been recognized for all of written history. It was first alluded to in 1553 B.C. by the Egyptian physician Hesy-Ra, who described it in ancient papyruses. The word "diabetes" was first used by the Greek physician, Aretaeus the Cappadocian (30–90 A.D.).[2] It was Aretaeus, as well, who first recognized type 2 diabetes as a separate entity; he called it "secondary diabetes." But he is better known for his colorful description of type 1:

> Diabetes is a wonderful affection, not very frequent among men, being a melting down of the flesh and limbs into urine. The patients never stop making water, but the flow is incessant, as if the opening of aqueducts. Life is short, disgusting, and painful; thirst unquenchable, excessive drinking, which, however, is disproportionate to the large quantity of urine; for more urine is passed, and one can not stop them from drinking or making water. Or if for a time they abstain from drinking, their mouth becomes parched and their body dry; the viscera seem as if scorched up; they are affected with nausea, restlessness and a burning thirst; and at no distant time they expire.

Another two thousand years went by before the actual metabolic distinctions between types 1 and 2 were defined. Sir Harold Percival Hinsworth of the University of London, writing in the British journal *The. Lancet,* clarified these differences in 1936. But it was only when the industrialization of America began to undermine our nutritional environment and remove our need to expend energy that the disease began to flourish as a side effect of our way of life.

The genetic potential to develop type 2 diabetes has been there all along, sleeping, if you will, ready to be awakened like a seed in the desert waiting for rain. You do not become a type 2 diabetic simply by chance; you must occupy a particular "pathological niche," a particular socioeconomic and nutritional environment tempered by a sedentary lifestyle. Here in the United States and throughout most of the world, through private enterprise and endless advertising, we have created food choices and energy saving devices that overwhelm the limits of personal restraint. A mere 10 percent of our supermarket food is natural. The rest has been altered; tainted with artificial coloring, flavor enhancers, preservatives, or infused fat, or sugar coated to appeal to the eye, the tastebuds, and our pocketbooks. Our food supply is no longer fresh, nutritious, and healthful. It has been converted to a health risk, a nutritional booby trap, one that leads to obesity and type 2 diabetes. Though we know what we eat has been altered to suit our tastes and please our appetites, most of us ignore the obvious health hazards. We consume it anyway.

That pathological niche in which type 2 diabetes thrives is rapidly expanding into a worldwide artificial environment. Annie Walker lives in that environment. She can not depend on the "family genes" to anticipate a long healthy life or, for that matter, predict a short one. Indeed, no one can. Today, the environment plays too big a role. Once a condition thought to be limited to poor overweight people, today type 2 diabetes affects every color, every race, and every class. And our American diet and lack of exercise is certainly not the only cause. The disease may be the result of a "genetic overload," a pancreatic affliction, a metabolic response to pregnancy, the side effect of a medication, the acquisition of a "risk-gene," a spinoff of a pre-existing disease, or the deleterious effects of aging upon insulin. As we go through life, it appears that what we eat and how much we exercise can influence the very structure and function of our DNA. Our individual genetic blueprints are not as stable as we thought. Our genes, we shall see, can be altered mid-stream, as we live, by our environment. And, incredibly, in some cases, the expression of these changed genes may be passed, like blue eyes, from generation to generation.

Though the environment plays the biggest role, occasionally an individual with no apparent risk factors will develop the disease. But make no mistake; the flawed, fundamental link between our modern post-industrial way of life and our ancient genetic makeup is ultimately responsible for this scourge.

Some people are born with a greater genetic potential to develop type 2 diabetes. There are, however, mitigating factors. Some of us inherit obesity-promoting genes that lead to type 2 diabetes (over 300 have been identified). Unfortunately, many of us are unaware of the dire, longterm consequences of how we live and what we eat. Your parents' generation had the genes for type 2 diabetes, but they were dormant; now they're awake and playing havoc with our insulin metabolism. The socioeconomic environment, the pathological niche for type 2 diabetes is in place. We've replaced our natural environment with an artificial one that is incompatible with healthy living and has begun to lower life expectancy and overburden our healthcare system.

According to the Centers for Disease Control (CDC) and the National Institute of Health (NIH), 33 percent of today's American children will, at some point in their lives, develop type 2 diabetes. Ethnicity is an important factor. The genetic makeup and lifestyles of different ethnic groups assure that 50 percent of Hispanic children, 50 percent of African-American children, and 75 percent of Native American children will develop diabetes. On average, the uninformed diabetic's life expectancy will be reduced by about 20 years. For the educated, however, the onset of type 2 diabetes can be delayed or completely avoided, and, for those already afflicted, lifestyle changes can limit the number of complications, or at least minimize their intensity. Advances in modern medical know-how, technology, and pharmaceuticals has extended the life expectancy of the pre-fast food generation, middle-aged and older Americans, but in the process has created a paradox — the opportunity for them, too, to develop type 2 diabetes.

Have we outsmarted ourselves? Over the millennia, humans have developed complex brains. We have a uniquely superior ability to think and reason; we no longer depend on innate biological mechanisms like hibernation, cold-bloodedness, specialized physiology, and risk-taking in order to survive harsh times. Our instinct for self preservation has been commandeered by our larger brains. Modern man depends on common sense, reasoning and education. But we have limitations, gaps in our ability to reason and compute; we are not good at reasoning based on probability. Sometimes, indeed often, we know the possible consequences of our actions, but we ignore them in favor of instant gratification. We willingly take risks.

Psychologists consider risk-taking a personality trait. Some of us accept the probability of a harmful event occurring as a result of our actions, especially when that harmful event is delayed or not immediately apparent. When we take a risk with immediate consequences, say sky diving, we experience a physiologic reaction — rapid heart rate, sweating, and apprehension. These reactions may keep us on the ground, but we get no such physiologic reaction when the risks are not obvious (or camouflaged by unscrupulous advertising), or if the consequences are delayed.

Tens of thousands of years ago, in order to survive in an untamed world we were gradually programmed. We evolved to fit, to mesh, like all species, with our environment. The biological blueprints for evolution are drawn by the environment, and human evolution — the gradual construction of our genetic makeup — is glacially slow. Our ancient genetic makeup persists today, but we, "smart man," have altered our environment. We've swiftly changed it from natural to artificial. Our genes, however, have not caught up. They are out of sync with the health risks of our new environment. We live in a different world, an industrialized world. We still defy danger. We must. Risk-taking is part of our ancient genetic makeup. For many, the health risks of today's diet and lifestyle go unheeded or unrecognized. And for others, caution is suppressed by the invincible mindset of youth.

Most of us recognize the problem, but will we voluntarily change our eating habits? It's not likely. In view of the healthcare crisis resulting from obesity and type 2 diabetes, specifically its burden on government healthcare expenditure, many local governments are attempting to address the problem. In New York City restaurants, the use of harmful, artery-clogging hydrogenated fats for cooking is now punishable by a hefty fine. New York state government, facing a budget shortfall, is suggesting an obesity tax, adding a few cents to the cost of sugary soft drinks. In San Francisco the local government is considering placing limits on the number of fast food restaurants per square mile. When Oklahoma City was designated by *Men's Fitness* magazine as one of the nation's fattest cities, Mick Cornett, its overweight mayor, was inspired to challenge his constituents to join him in a citywide weight loss and exercise program.[3] The goal: to lose 1 million pounds in one year. A Web site (www.thiscityisgoingonadiet.com) was set up to inspire and assist obese Okies to shed weight and become fit. Oklahoma ranks fourth in its percentage of type 2 diabetics nationally. There is pressure by health-conscious groups to require chain restaurants to list nutritional facts on their menus. School lunch menus are changing, there is a push to reinstitute physical education classes, and our government is allotting funds to promote healthy living (a pittance when compared to the fast food industry's advertising budget). And, of course, nutritional charts are printed on packaged goods, but they are often misleading and difficult to interpret.

Research involving the genetics of diabetes is progressing worldwide.

Perhaps, in time, a genetic intervention may eliminate types 1 and 2 diabetes. However, until that happens, the incidence of type 2 diabetes with its inevitable complications heart disease, kidney failure, peripheral artery disease, amputation, stroke and neuropathy will continue to rise. Many diabetic complications can be avoided or minimized with proper self-care, but when they do appear they must be dealt with, and that is often the job of the surgeon. Diabetes is not generally thought of as a surgical disease. The initial diagnosis, everyday care, medications, diet, insulin regulation, lifestyle guidance and medical advice are dispensed by the endocrinologist, the internist, or the family physician. The surgeon, however, is the one best equipped to handle the complications of diabetes mellitus. And now with the new specialty of metabolic surgery, in some cases, type 2 diabetes can be cured (see Chapter 3).

My intention in this book is to explain why type 2 diabetes has become so common, and to share the knowledge I've gained through 35 years of surgical experience in treating its grave, life-shortening complications. Sadly, most experts agree that for humanity as a whole it is already too late; the disease is out of control. But the enlightening information that follows will enable some fated-to-be type 2 diabetics to avoid the disease, and others to minimize or at least correctly treat its formidable complications.

Part One

The Social and Scientific Basis of Diabetes

Chapter 1

THE NEWLY DIAGNOSED DIABETIC: THE CASE OF GARY LUTTON

The heart of any large hospital is the emergency room — a way station for the human condition, where the sick and injured arrive by foot, car, ambulance or helicopter. Night and day, they pour through our emergency room doors as if arriving on a morbid, endless conveyor belt. Our E.R. has grown with the hospital, expanding five times since I began practice in the early 1970s. Today there are no empty beds. The halls are lined with moaning patients, heart monitor alarms are sounding, phones are ringing, and the waiting room is standing room only. Red flashing ambulance lights blink through the glass sliding doors. We're not in a war zone. There is no pandemic, no local disaster. The onslaught results from the myriad diseases, defects, infections and trauma to which mankind is subjected. In most cases the malady seems unavoidable: appendicitis, ruptured aneurysms, ectopic pregnancies, automobile accidents — there's no end to the list.

In some cases, however, the reason for the E.R. visit is unwittingly self-inflicted, the result of an inappropriate or perhaps unavoidable lifestyle. In some cases the expression of a latent hereditary defect brings people in, a genetic flaw, or an epigenetic phenomenon — a gene that is expressed only when combined with a specific lifestyle. Type 2 diabetes is such a disease. "Type 2 diabetes." It sounds innocuous enough, however with its many life- and limb-threatening complications, it has become the scourge of the twenty-first century.

Over the last few decades, because of its greatly increasing incidence, type 2 diabetes has been described as an epidemic. Epidemics, however, are self-limited; they go away. Type 2 diabetes is actually an *endemic* disease. It prevails continually in most of the civilized world. Unlike an epidemic, it won't run its course. It is appearing earlier in life, lasting longer, and is causing dire physical complications. Diabetes is the major cause for amputations, kidney failure, and blindness in the United States. Heart disease is four times more common among diabetics and strokes are twice as common. These are a few of the complications treated by the surgeon — yet preventable by an enlightened public.[1]

A Typical Onset

Gary Lutton had been in the emergency room for nearly five hours when the E.R. physician called me back to the hospital. His incessant trips to the bathroom worried his wife, and when he told her his belly had begun to ache, she diagnosed a urinary tract infection. That's what prompted the visit. The E.R. staff did the usual workup — a complete blood count, blood chemistries, and a chest X-ray. The real diagnosis came quickly. His blood sugar level was 502. Normal is less than 120. That single blood test was enough. Gary was diabetic. At first the E.R. doctor thought that was Gary's only problem — new onset diabetes — but when he saw Gary grimace whenever he moved, the doctor decided he'd play it safe; he ordered a CAT scan. The report came back: Acute perforated appendicitis. "A text-book picture," the radiologist said. That's why they called me in — to remove Gary's appendix.

I found him in bed number 14, his wife, Louise, at his bedside. I began to introduce myself when she interrupted. "Oh, you must be the diabetes doctor."

"No," I told her. "I'm not an internist or an endocrinologist. I'm a surgeon. I treat the complications of diabetes."

"Appendicitis isn't a diabetic disease," she said.

"That's right," I agreed. "Your husband is a diabetic with appendicitis and the combination requires an altered approach to the usual treatment."

During my thirty-five years of practice I've occupied a unique surgical niche. I've developed a relationship with many diabetologists, who, in view of my experience with operating on diabetics, often refer their patients when it appears they require surgery. They know that diabetics have an increased risk of complications, even death, when compared to nondiabetic patients. And, unfortunately, because diabetics often develop surgical complications unique to their disease, they're far more likely to require surgery than non-diabetics.

I explained to Mrs. Lutton that diabetics are subject to the same surgical diseases as non-diabetics. Diabetes, of course, creates its own array of surgical conditions, but this wasn't the time to discuss that. I explained to her that the care of diabetics before, during and after the surgery differs from that of nondiabetics. Blood sugar must be closely monitored, cardiovascular status carefully evaluated, and surgical techniques modified to assure healing and reduce the chances of residual or postoperative infection.

I looked Gary over. He was lying still, a whale of a man. He covered most of the cot. As I began to examine him, his wife piped up. "We didn't even know he was a diabetic till half an hour ago!" I explained that many type 2 diabetics go through a pre-diabetic phase; a period of years before a symptom appears. This silent phase might be uncovered inadvertently by simple blood tests, or wisely tested for by an alert physician. And some people, Mr. Lutton for one, may be overtly diabetic without recognizing it. But, inevitably, some stressful situation appears and exposes the condition. In his case the acute infection, the appendicitis, drove his blood sugar up and made the diagnosis unmistakable. Had he not gotten appendicitis, he may have gone undiagnosed even longer and, without treatment, risked early complications.

He looked sick. His face was flushed, his breathing rapid, and his legs were drawn up to ease his belly ache. In spite of a 101°F fever, his skin was dry. He wasn't sweating, not unusual when the blood sugar is high. With diabetes, sweating comes when the blood sugar drops. His pulse rate was 90, respirations 16 per minute, and his lungs were clear. His enormous abdomen heaved with each breath; it overlapped his groins and hid a red, fungal rash. Despite the protruding belly, his arms and legs were not heavy. He had what's called "central obesity," a SpongeBob body type, a common finding in type 2 diabetics. His wife kept talking as I examined him, but Gary remained silent — until I got to his belly. I pressed lightly on his right lower abdomen. His expression didn't change. "Does that hurt?" I asked.

"A little," he said. Then I pulled my hand quickly from his abdomen, letting the tissues rebound. He winced. "That hurt." His response to this maneuver showed me that his infection had been brewing for a while, perhaps days. It indicated that the sensitive, inner lining of his abdominal wall, the peritoneum over his appendix, was inflamed, a sure sign of infection within the abdomen — peritonitis. A nondiabetic patient, one with normal pain sensation, would have noticed his problem sooner, much sooner. Appendicitis is more severe in diabetics. They don't feel the pain as intensely as nondiabetics. And to add to the delay, overweight patients "wall off" their infected appendix; they insulate it with intra-abdominal fat which has no nerves. So for Mr. Lutton to show up already ruptured, but with few complaints, was no surprise.

Louise Lutton, aware of the CAT scan findings, asked when we would operate. I told her we needed time to hydrate her husband with IV fluids and retest his blood sugar. If it remained high, he would need more insulin to bring it down. She looked down at her husband, then back up at me. Her eyes were wet. She needed reassurance. I took her to the E.R. lounge. "Once we get him rehydrated," I told her, "when his appendix is out, and the infection drained, his blood sugar will go back down. In the long run," I said, "he might not need insulin — maybe not even pills. Hopefully, he'll be able to control his diabetes with diet and exercise." Now, away from the bedside, she told me his dad was diabetic and died in his 60s, two years after losing two toes. I explained that type 2 diabetes may be genetic and that at least one third of us carry the genes. "If the conditions are right," I said

"What conditions?" she asked.

"Lifestyle conditions, his eating habits and exercise routine."

"He eats what he wants and he sits at a desk."

"I know," I said. "And to some extent that's why he's got diabetes, but that can be controlled." She helped me fill in the history: two sons, ages 12 and 14. He took blood pressure medications, weighed 244 pounds, and hadn't seen a doctor in six years.

I pulled the surgical consent form from the chart and went over the risks and possible complications. I explained that she'd have to sign it instead of Gary because the E.R. doctor had given him morphine. She did. She knew I wasn't basing the need for surgery on the CAT scan findings alone. I had intentionally demonstrated the physical findings of peritonitis — the rebound tenderness. She saw him wince.

It is important that the patient and family fully understand and accept without question the need for surgery. In a case like this, the CAT scan findings should not be the only reason to operate. I, too, needed the proof provided by the physical examination. The last thing I want is to operate based solely on an X-ray interpretation, and later, in the O.R., discover that the X-ray had been misread. Sometimes out-of-control diabetics come to the E.R. with abdominal pain that has no surgical basis, and occasionally CAT scans are misinterpreted.

I called the operating room to schedule him, called anesthesia for a pre-op evaluation, and paged the surgical resident to come down, look him over, and complete the paperwork. The resident sent Sanjieve, the intern. We went over the blood work and reviewed the history. The repeated blood sugar test had fallen to 180. The insulin was working. The Foley catheter, inserted earlier by an E.R. nurse, was draining copious, clear, urine. He was rehydrated. I slowed the IV rate to 125 cc per hour, reassured Mr. Lutton, and introduced Louise to Sanjieve and to the nurse who would take her to the O.R. waiting area. I'd see her there as soon as we finished. I told her to try not to worry; we'd take care of Gary. Then we walked down the hall to the radiology suite and stood behind the radiologist as he reviewed Mr. Lutton's CAT scan for us. He pointed to the frame showing the appendix in cross-section. It was more than one centimeter wide, surrounded by foamy fat that was peppered with tiny, black air bubbles, and it sat in a puddle of fluid with the consistency of pus. The appendix is not always in the same spot; it may be low in the pelvis or, in late pregnancy, high up in the belly just under the gall bladder. Mr. Lutton's appendix was deep in his pelvis, perched on his psoas, the long, fat cylindrical muscle adjacent to the spine. (It's familiar to butchers because, in cattle, the tender psoas muscle is filet mignon.)

Gary Lutton's Operation

At 2 A.M. we were in the O.R. It was quiet, with only one other case going on. Nelly, the night-shift nurse, pointed down the hall and yawned, "You're in room eleven; they're ready for you." I explained to Frank, the first-year resident who'd arrived to assist, that considering the physical findings and the CAT scan picture of an already-ruptured appendicitis, we'd operate through an open incision, not laparoscopically. That would be quicker, I told him, and allow us to stay right over the ruptured appendix. We'd avoid the risk of seeding the rest of his belly with pus.

Dr. Noon, the anesthesiologist, put Gary to sleep, slipped in the endotracheal tube, and attached Gary to the respirator. With the patient on the operating table and under anesthesia, and with the muscle relaxant medication in effect, I re-examined his flaccid abdomen. Now, despite his obesity, I could feel the fist-sized, firm, inflammatory mass encasing his infected appendix. I asked Frank to feel it. Now we knew exactly where to make our incision.

Janet is the circulating nurse, the only one in the room who is not "sterile." She wears a mask, but no sterile gloves. She can touch what we can't, mop our brows, and adjust the lights. She's the link between us and the supply cabinets, the telephone, and the blood bank. She shaved Gary's abdomen, scrubbed him with a soapy sponge, and blotted his belly dry with a towel. Then Laura, the scrub nurse, painted his abdomen with a coat of brown Betadine antiseptic.

Frank and I went to scrub. We watched through the glass as Laura draped Gary's belly with sterile, green towels and laparotomy sheets. Then she handed us our gowns and pulled on our gloves. Frank stood opposite me with Mr. Lutton sandwiched between us. I checked with Dr. Noon, he nodded that we could start. Laura handed me the scalpel. I made a transverse incision, about three inches long, through the skin of Mr. Lutton's right lower abdomen, just over the palpable inflammatory mass. I cut carefully down through 4 inches of subcutaneous fat to the fascia, the tough fibrous covering of the external oblique and rectus abdominis muscles. I opened the fascia with my scalpel and, using a clamp, spread the two muscles apart. No significant bleeding. I tied off, and then divided a pulsating branch of the inferior epigastric artery with its adjacent vein. This exposed the pearly, peritoneal lining of the abdominal cavity. Usually paper thin, his peritoneum was thickened, inflamed by the infection beneath it. I opened it with my scalpel, inserted most of my hand and, with my index finger deep in his belly, looped his swollen appendix. Surgeons' fingers have eyes. I eased his appendix into view. The last two inches were black — gangrenous. I lined the walls of the incision with sterile pads. I maneuvered a Babcock clamp between loops of bowel, gently grasped the swollen, decomposing appendix, and eased it up, taking care not to rip it from the cecum. The foul stench of days-old infection forced Frank's head back. I pinched the triangular veil of fatty tissue that holds the appendix to the cecum and, in it, felt the pulsating appendicle artery. I clamped the vessel, and then tied it off with a cat gut suture. Then I looped the base of the appendix with a cat gut ligature, cinched the three knots down, and cut it off. All that remained was the tied appendicle stump, sitting on the cecum like the end of a pink party balloon.

Still in the gentle jaws of the Babcock clamp, I handed the rotting, black tissue to Laura. "No doubt about this one," she said, as she opened the clamp and dropped it into a specimen jar. We cultured the wound, irrigated with sterile saline and suctioned the area in the pelvis where pus had accumulated. Then we placed a soft, rubber Penrose drain in the empty abscess cavity. We changed our gloves and closed the belly, layer by layer, with absorbable suture. Finally, we irrigated the subcutaneous tissue, changed to clean gloves, and closed the skin loosely with blue nylon sutures. Frank tied the knots. "Not tight, Frank, you don't want to cut off the blood supply to the skin edge. That kills the cells and feeds the infection."

Frank glanced at the specimen jar. The room stank from pus. He wondered aloud why the patient hadn't come in sooner. I explained again — diabetics simply don't feel pain as intensely as nondiabetics. Their sensory nerves are damaged. And the abundant visceral fat pad of overweight patients insulates the inflammatory process, further blunting the pain. It's as if their early-warning system has shorted out. We sewed the floppy, yellow latex drain to his skin and made it "nurse-proof." Now secure, it couldn't be pulled out inadvertently during a hasty dressing change, or be sucked back into his belly with a deep breath. As we placed the last stitch, as if on cue, Gary gagged and opened his eyes. We bandaged the incision. Dr. Noon glanced at the oxygen sensor, disconnected the respirator, and watched Gary breathe. Then, satisfied with the vital signs, he removed the endotracheal tube. The five of us lifted the patient onto the gurney and wheeled him down the hall to the recovery room.

I went over the written postoperative orders with his recovery room nurse. Then I walked down the hall to the surgical waiting area, quiet at 3:30 A.M. and empty, except for pink-and puffy-eyed Louise. "Gary's doing fine," I told her,. "And the recovery room's not busy, so in about thirty minutes, when he's more awake, his nurse will come get you." She thanked me, and with a quiver, said, "I'm worried — the diabetes and all."

I told her what I believe is true: that one way to live a long life is to contract a chronic disease like diabetes and nurse it into old age. I left the waiting area, thinking that your fate is really in your genes. They determine so much more than we realize, including, in a surreptitious way, what diseases we get and how well we can handle them. Diabetes, types 1 and 2, each have their genetic roots. The internist can try to control the disease, the surgeon can handle most of the complications, but education is the key to prevention and scientific research the path to cure.

Gary Lutton's Case — Morning Rounds

I was back at 7 A.M. for morning rounds with the intern and residents. We discussed Gary Lutton's case. I explained to Sanjieve that type 2 diabetes may exist in a sub-clinical, non–apparent state for years during, which the patient may attribute fatigue to overwork, and frequent urination to an enlarged prostate or a weak bladder. Sooner or later though, some stressful situation will drive the blood sugar up. It may be appendicitis, an ingrown toenail, too many jelly doughnuts, a cold — anything! A simple blood test will reveal the high glucose; a urinalysis may show sugar in the urine and the diagnosis is established.

I told Sanjieve, who was from India, that he was fortunate to have been born at the right time. Two thousand years ago young Hindu physicians were obliged to taste their patients' urine to detect the sweetness and make the diagnosis of diabetes.[2] They were called "water tasters." Frank added that in parts of Africa, rural Madagascar to be precise, folk healers to this day, use primitive methods of diagnosis. When a healer suspects his patient is diabetic, he takes him into the bush, leads him near an ant hill, and asks him to urinate. If there's sugar in his urine, the ants are attracted and swarm over it. They'll be repelled, though, by the unsweetened urine of a nondiabetic.[3] Today, in most of the world, simple blood tests are used. If two random fasting glucose tests show a level of 120 or higher, then the diagnosis is made.

Diabetes mellitus types 1 and 2 share common symptoms and complications, but stem from different insulin defects. In type 1, there is an absolute lack of insulin, the result of the destruction of insulin-producing, pancreatic beta cells by the patient's own immune system. Type 1 diabetes is a genetically linked, non-preventable disease. It is thought (by some investigators) to be induced by injury to the beta cells, perhaps as a result of an intrauterine or early childhood viral infection, like measles, mumps or Coxsackie virus.

Type 2 diabetes, on the other hand, is the result of an individual's inability to use the normal insulin that his pancreatic beta cells secrete. As time passes, type 2s develop insufficient production of insulin as well. So type 2 diabetics have two metabolic defects: insulin resistance, the inability of insulin to carry glucose from the bloodstream into the cells (its primary function) and a progressive inability of the pancreas to produce insulin.

Approximately 80 to 90 percent of diabetics are type 2. The rest, 10 to 20 percent, are type 1. Type 1 diabetics are sometimes called juvenile diabetics or early-onset diabetics because their disease starts in childhood. Type 1 diabetics are absolutely dependent upon self-injected, pharmacologic insulin. They have none, or too little of their own. Many type 2 diabetics eventually become dependent on injectable insulin as well. The sugar-lowering pills they take tend to lose their effectiveness, and insulin production from their own beta cells dwindles as the years go by.

The Many Forms of Diabetes Mellitus

Old ideas persist. Patients and many doctors still think of diabetes simply as "type 1" or "type 2." Generally speaking the pathologic basis for type 1 diabetes is an inability of the pancreatic beta cells to produce insulin, whereas type 2 diabetics can produce insulin, but it is ineffective, and eventually production is diminished as well. But there are actually a number of varieties of each type, many of which have surfaced in recent years. Subtle differences in these subtypes may require altered treatments, a fact not always recognized by the physician or the patient.

One such variety, often misdiagnosed as type 2 because of its late onset and initial good response to oral medications, is called latent autoimmune diabetes in the adult (LADA). Unlike typical type 1 diabetics, individuals with this variety are usually diagnosed after age 30. Obesity, defined by the American Heart Association as having a waist circumference of 40 inches (103 cm) or greater in a male, or 34 inches (88 cm) or greater in a female, is not a prerequisite. Early on, patients with LADA are not insulin dependent; they can get by with diet control and oral hypoglycemic drugs for up to three years. Eventually though, when enough of their beta cells have been destroyed by their own immune system, all latent type 1 diabetics become insulin dependent.

Research in England suggests that about 10 percent of adults with diabetes have LADA. Latent type 1 diabetes is not a consequence of lifestyle. As with most varieties of diabetes it has genetic roots. This type of diabetes appears later in life because the destruction of the beta cells in the pancreas occurs more slowly than with typical, early-onset type 1 diabetes. The diagnosis of LADA is made in the clinical laboratory with blood tests designed to reveal the presence of islet cell antibodies, just as with the more common early-onset type 1 diabetes.

For the newly diagnosed diabetic, consultation with a specialist is important. Many diabetic patients would benefit from the specialized care of an endocrinologist or diabetologist, but have no access to diabetologists; instead, they're treated by internists or primary care physicians. The field of endocrinology requires specialty training, is work intensive, and is financially unattractive. There's little incentive for medical students to pursue it. In 2006, the entire state of New Jersey turned out only four certifiable endocrinologists. Islet cell antibody testing (the glutamic acid decarboxylase autoantibody or GADA test), for example, is infrequently ordered by the non-diabetologist/endocrinologist. This test may be of value for some adults presumed to have type 2 diabetes, as it would help differentiate them from LADA-type 1 diabetics, who often require insulin early on.[4] In other words, often stereotyped, obese, non diet-conscious, sedentary, type 2 diabetics may be misdiagnosed. They may actually be latent type 1 diabetics. And in order to better control their blood sugars and avoid complications, they may benefit from the early institution of insulin therapy. Fortunately LADA is relatively rare and some physicians who deal regularly with diabetics classify them accurately using routine clinical and laboratory testing.

So far, we have discussed three, genetically-based varieties of diabetes mellitus. They are:

(1) Type 1, genetic in origin, but thought to be triggered by some sort of common, early in life viral infection. It is characterized by insulin dependence, frequent swings in blood sugar levels and is not associated with lifestyle choices.

(2) Type 2, often genetically mediated, but not characterized by frequent swings in blood sugar levels. In the majority of cases it is associated with an unhealthy lifestyle and often progresses to insulin dependence after eight to ten years.

(3) Latent autoimmune diabetes in the adult (LADA), a variant of type 1 diabetes that comes about later in life and may easily be misdiagnosed as type 2 diabetes, particularly if the patient is overweight.

A fourth variety of genetically induced diabetes mellitus is called maturity onset diabetes of the young (MODY). This relatively uncommon type of diabetes (less than 3 percent) is the result of a rare, single-gene mutation which is inherited in autosomal dominant fashion.[5] In other words, it's passed down from generation to generation in a predictable fashion. If your mother or father has it, you will have a fifty percent chance of inheriting it. To date, MODY is the only variety of diabetes in which a specific, single gene defect has been clearly isolated. Consequently, MODY is the only type of diabetes for which specific genetic testing can be used to make the diagnosis.[6] Six single-gene variants of MODY have been identified. With MODY the genetic mutation causes impaired release or decreased production of insulin by the pancreatic beta cells.

A review of the medical literature indicates that MODY is given more attention in Europe where genetic testing is routinely used to make the diagnosis. European medicine puts greater emphasis on prevention. In the U.S. preventive medicine takes a back seat. The emphasis is placed on treatment. It's simply more profitable. American primary care practitioners are overburdened. They deal with so wide a variety of diseases, they may not be familiar with the multiple types of diabetes. To the busy physician, MODY looks a lot like type 1, but unlike type 1, it does not necessarily require insulin injections, because oral medications are just as effective.[7] Genetic testing is rarely done here, but it should be used when MODY is suspected because it not only leads to proper treatment, it identifies potentially afflicted family members before they become symptomatic.

The Pancreas and Insulin Metabolism

The pancreas sits smack in the middle of the human body. It's shaped like a fish with its head inextricably fused to the duodenum. Its tail is sheathed in large, flimsy blood vessels and cupped in the crotch of the spleen, while its body lies over the spine, sandwiched between the stomach above and the pulsating aorta and fragile vena cava below. The bile duct snakes right through its head, and the formidable blood supply to the liver and intestinal tract, the portal vein and the mesenteric vessels, pass through the gland marking the surgical junction between its body and head. The pancreas can be a surgical nightmare. (See figs. 1, 2.)

Most glands are either *exocrine* or *endocrine*. The pancreas is both. Exocrine glands produce fluids or enzymes that are secreted through ducts directly into the gastrointestinal tract or body surface. Enzymes are chemical catalysts, protein compounds that induce chemical changes in other substances. The pancreas manufactures digestive enzymes (pancreatic juice) and, in response to the presence of food in the stomach and first portion of the small intestine, secretes these enzymes directly into the gastrointestinal tract, where they dissolve swallowed food, breaking it into molec-

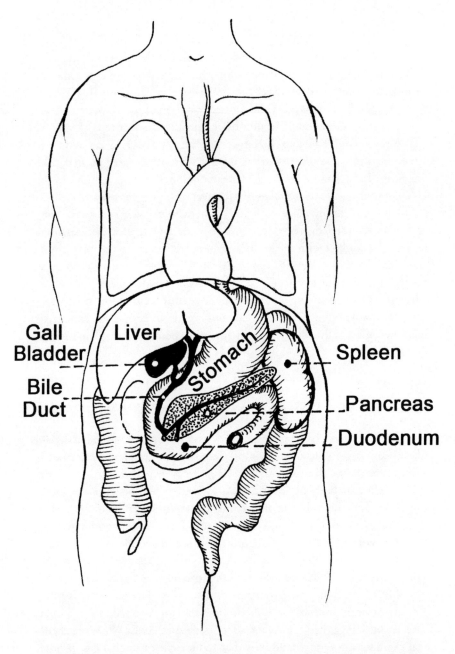

Gall Bladder

Liver

Stomach

Spleen

Bile Duct

Pancreas

Duodenum

Fig. #1: Pancreas. The pancreas, with its insulin-secreting islets, is shaped like a fish. Its head, pierced by the bile duct, is fused to the duodenum. Its body, atop the aorta and vena cava, is sandwiched between the stomach and the spine, and its tail is buried in the spleen. The entire gland is wrapped in blood vessels, large and small.

The Pancreas Depicted Without
the Overlying Stomach

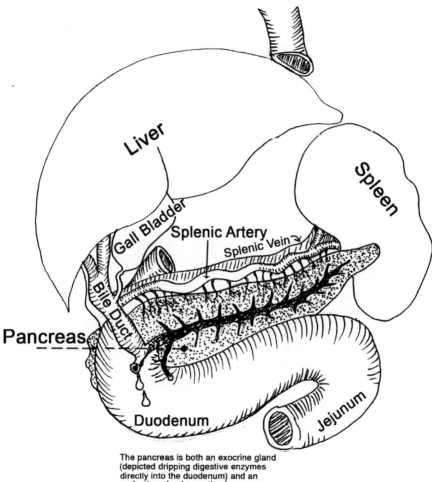

The pancreas is both an exocrine gland
(depicted dripping digestive enzymes
directly into the duodenum) and an
endocrine gland secreting hormones
insulin and glucagon directly into the
bloodstream.

Fig. #2: The pancreas, two glands in one structure. A closeup view shows the
bile duct joining the pancreatic duct to form one channel, which carries a
mix of bile from the liver and pancreatic enzymes directly into the duodenum. This is the exocrine portion of the gland. The islets of Langerhans (little black dots) are the endocrine portion; they release insulin directly into
the bloodstream.

ular particles. These molecular nutrients are then taken into the blood-stream and transported to where they are needed for tissue growth or repair, or stored and used as fuel for energy, as in the case of sugar. Other examples of exocrine glands are sweat, tear, and salivary glands.

Endocrine glands, on the other hand, secrete their hormones directly into the bloodstream. A hormone is a "chemical messenger," a substance produced in one organ and carried via the bloodstream to another organ that it sets into motion. About 10,000 islands of specialized cells make up the endocrine portion of the pancreas. These islands are randomly scattered throughout the pancreas like blueberries in a muffin. Together they are called the islets of Langerhans. Within the 10,000 islands (the "islets") are the beta cells. These cells are genetically programmed to synthesize the hormone insulin, which is released directly into the bloodstream in response to high blood sugar levels. The pituitary gland, the ovary, and the thyroid are other examples of endocrine glands.

Paul Langerhans, a German anatomist working in the late 1800s, discovered the islets, but he never knew their function. Many scientists suspected the pancreas was, in some way, responsible for glucose metabolism. Their suspicions were confirmed by accident, as often happens with scientific discoveries, when in 1899 the European researchers Minkowski and von Mering removed the pancreas of a dog and noted a few days later that flies were feeding on the dog's urine. They tested the urine and found sugar. Following this discovery several European scientists independently identified the mysterious islets as the source. They laid the groundwork for the Canadian scientist Frederick Banting and his student Charles Best who, in 1922, were the first to isolate and use insulin to successfully treat a type 1 diabetic patient.

Insulin is not a one-trick hormone; it's multifunctional. One function is to escort glucose (sugar) from the bloodstream into the cells of the body where it can be used as a source of fuel for energy; it acts as a key that allows glucose (sugar) to exit the bloodstream and enter certain cells of the body. A second function is to aid in the clearance of lipids (fat) from the blood and promote its storage in adipose tissue. Insulin also plays an important role in protein synthesis. When insulin is absent (type 1) or if the "key" doesn't work (type 2, insulin resistance), the blood sugar levels remain high. And high blood sugar, of course, is the classic laboratory finding that defines all types of diabetes mellitus.

All life is a chemical balancing act. Insulin, like many life sustaining hormones, has a counterpart, an antagonist — a hormone called glucagon.

Glucagon, like insulin, is manufactured in the islets of the pancreas, in the alpha cells. After insulin transfers glucose directly from the bloodstream into the liver, it is converted into long sugar chains, storage units called glycogen. When the blood sugar is low, or no food is available, glycogen is metabolized back into simple sugar and moved by glucagon directly into the bloodstream. From there it is escorted into the cells by insulin and used as fuel for energy. In the non-diabetic these two hormones act in concert to keep your blood sugar in the normal range, between 60 and 100 mg/dL (fasting).

In the diabetic, the balance between insulin and glucagon is out of kilter; too much glucagon keeps blood sugars high. Scientists have been anxious to learn exactly how to turn glucagon off, for that would provide another way, a treatment, to lower the glucose levels of out-of-control diabetics. After decades of trying, they've come up empty.[8] Mother Nature, on the other hand, has found the antidote to glucagon. It grows on trees. Specifically, Ackee trees. Originally found in tropical West Africa, the Ackee tree thrives in many tropical countries, but it is famous in Jamaica. But all is not perfect in paradise. Eaten before it ripens, the Ackee fruit's nutritious, soft, white meat will make you sick. It contains hypoglycin A, a potent glucagon antagonist that causes Jamaican vomiting sickness, characterized by a potentially fatal, dangerously-low blood sugar. As the fruit ripens, the hypoglycin A turns into a harmless chemical. Painful experience has taught humans to avoid unripe Ackee fruit, but tropical birds need no lesson; instinctively aware of the fatal side effects, they ignore the unripe fruit.

The pancreas is not unique to humans. All vertebrates possess a pancreas, hence they all can develop diabetes when subjected to pancreatic damage (environmental or otherwise). Many animal species suffer diseases that are similar to human illnesses. For example, cats get leukemia, dogs are subject to arthritis of the hip joints, turtles can die from cardiac arrhythmias, and genetically altered rats are used as the animal model for diabetes research. Birds, though, are unique. When they develop diabetes, the symptoms are the same as in humans — frequent urination, excessive thirst, and the potential for organ, blood vessel, and nerve damage. But diabetes in birds is not caused by too little or malfunctioning insulin; the cause is too much glucagon.

The human pancreas, housing two glands in the same structure, occasionally trips over itself.[9] A disease of the exocrine portion may affect the endocrine portion (the islets) and result in yet another variety of diabetes, pancreatic or type 3c diabetes. Pancreatitis (a severe, sometimes fatal inflammation of the pancreas from gallstones, alcoholism, or very high blood lipid levels) and advanced cancer of the pancreas destroy pancreatic tissue, including the islets. The result is type 3c diabetes. Sometimes, seemingly unrelated diseases have as a spin-off temporary or permanent type 3c diabetes. Polycystic ovary syndrome affects one in ten women and is one such disease. This syndrome is characterized anatomically by abnormally large ovaries studded with multiple, fluid-filled cysts. Afflicted women are typically overweight, don't ovulate, and have excess body hair. Occasionally they have male pattern baldness, grow multiple tiny skin tags, experience bloating and abdominal cramps, and are plagued by mood swings (PMS). They develop high blood pressure and elevated cholesterol, and their metabolism is beset by insulin resistance, the physiologic defect responsible for type 2 diabetes.

Cystic fibrosis is caused by an inheritable genetic mutation; it affects 30,000 people in the United States. Worldwide, it affects primarily Europeans and Ashkenazi Jews, but anyone can develop it. Cystic fibrosis affects the glandular structures throughout the body, causing them to produce thickened secretions which disrupt the transfer of body fluids. These thickened fluids clog the air passages in the lungs, causing pneumonia, and block the pancreatic ducts, causing severe pancreatic inflammation, pancreatitis. This leads to destruction of the beta cells. Insulin production ceases, and the result is type 3c diabetes.

The relationship between schizophrenia and type 2 diabetes has been known for over a century. Studies indicate that more than 14 percent of schizophrenics over age forty are diabetic. Apparently the two diseases are genetically linked.[10] Moreover, recent research shows that certain anti-psychotic drugs have side effects which further increase the incidence of diabetes in the schizophrenic population.

Several other commonly used medications cause diabetes as a side effect. Perhaps the most common drugs to cause type 2 diabetes are the corticosteroids. Prednisone is the most frequently used steroid. These anti-inflammatory medications treat a variety of conditions, from asthma to rheumatoid arthritis. They cause type 2 diabetes by increasing abdominal obesity with its associated insulin resistance, a side effect seen with other drugs as well. The outlook for AIDS-infected patients has improved dramatically; that is, if the patient can afford the antiretroviral medications (c-ART) required to treat the disease.[11] These drugs often extend the AIDS patient's life, free of major complications, for decades. But few drugs come with no strings attached. These life-prolonging antiretroviral medications have a side effect similar to prednisone — the appearance of metabolic disorders. Type 2 diabetes is one of them. After six or seven years of treatment, an AIDS patient's chances of becoming diabetic are double that of the general population, and as the length of treatment with c-ART drugs increases, so do the chances of developing diabetes.

Aside from drugs, diseases, surgery, genes, and the environment there are other, recently described causes of diabetes. Lithotripsy is a non-surgical method of turning kidney stones into painlessly passed sand. But nothing in medicine is without risk.[12] Apparently the beta cells in the pancreatic islets are easily damaged by the shock waves used to pulverize the stones. Decades after lithotripsy treatment, as a delayed side effect, people treated by this method were found to be developing diabetes at four times the rate of the general population.

Occasionally, already diabetic patients may develop pancreatic *exocrine* insufficiency. In this case, the diabetic's pancreatic digestive enzymes don't work. As a result, fat and proteins pass through the gastrointestinal tract undigested. Undigested food not only loses its nutritional value, it becomes a powerful laxative. The medical term for diarrhea from undigested fat is *steatorrhea*. Fortunately, pancreatic exocrine malfunction is easier to treat than type 3c diabetes. Steatorrhea is eliminated by taking digestive enzymes in pill form before each meal or snack. Sometimes if the surgeon, for one reason or another, removes part of or the entire pancreas, the result can be the appearance of both type 3c diabetes and pancreatic exocrine insufficiency. With the increasing incidence of pancreatic cancer and the damaging effect of alcoholic pancreatitis, these operations are becoming more common (Fig. #2).

Insulin, Protein Metabolism, and the HbA1c

Insulin is an extremely important anabolic (tissue building) hormone. One cannot live very long without it. Prior to 1922, when injectable insulin was made available by the pharmaceutical company Eli Lilly, the life expectancy of the type 1 diabetic was measured in days or weeks. Before insulin, the most effective treatment (at least temporarily) was to withhold food. Starvation. Today, diabetics are armed with an arsenal of medications, blood glucose testing devices, treatment manuals, and nutritional guides, all of which are designed to help them manage their condition.

Fortunately, diabetes is one of the few serious diseases that is controllable by both the physician and the patient. Your physician's job is to prescribe the proper medications for blood sugar regulation and blood pressure, cholesterol, and lipid (triglyceride) control; and he must monitor for prevention of kidney failure. To be effective, he must follow the guidelines of the American Diabetes Association. The patient's role, aside from following doctor's advice, is to be knowledgeable enough to avoid the many risks that will worsen or complicate his condition. The diabetic, the pre-diabetic, and the physician have a unique tool, an ace in the hole — the HbA1c test. This test measures how well the patient and the physician together are controlling the disease. The numerical value of the HbA1c represents a person's average blood sugar over the previous three months. The HbA1c is like a golf score; the lower the better.

Most people, doctors and patients alike, think of insulin as the sugar hormone. But insulin is much more than that; insulin is a multi-functional hormone. It plays a crucial role in complex protein production. *Glycosylation,* the attachment of glucose to amino acids (proteins) using insulin as the glue is an essential step in the synthesis of muscle mass, proper wound healing, and the formation of many solid and hollow organs. And enzymatic glycosylation is essential in the production of that most important, extremely complex, oxygen-carrying protein — hemoglobin.

Some protein synthesis, however, does not require enzymatic glycosylation. Instead these proteins are produced by a process called *nonenzymatic glycosylation* (no enzymes required). Hemoglobin A1c (HbA1c), or glycohemoglobin, is one such protein. The HbA1c molecule is different from the majority of oxygen-carrying hemoglobin molecules is that it has a glucose moiety attached to the end of it; thus the name: glycohemoglobin. Glycohemoglobin, GHb or HbA1c (all are the same) normally makes up about 4 percent of the total hemoglobin in our red blood cells. The remaining 96 percent does not contain that glucose moiety. All hemoglobin resides in the blood, so it can be measured easily. The percentage of HbA1c in a person's blood (that hemoglobin with the glucose attached) is directly related to one's ever-changing blood sugar (glucose) level. As we know, the lack of effective insulin in diabetics results in greatly elevated blood sugar levels. We also know that the lifespan of a red blood cell is 120 days. During those 120 days, the nonenzymatic glycosylation of hemoglobin — the production of glycohemoglobin (HbA1c)—takes place. So in diabetes, a lack of functioning insulin (and chronically high blood sugars) results in high HbA1c levels.

The red hemoglobin molecule is extremely complex, but not unique. Chlorophyll has almost the exact complex structure, but rather than housing an iron atom (Fe) at its center, green chlorophyll is built around a single magnesium (mg) atom. Hemoglobin clings to oxygen and delivers it to our tissues, while chlorophyll makes and releases it so we can breathe it in. This basic similarity between plant and animal is something to consider when pondering the origin of life. But this is another story and has nothing to do with diabetes.

Hemoglobin A1c, however, is quite relevant. What follows is a brief history of its discovery. The separtion of this variety of hemoglobin from other forms was made by Huisman and Meycring in 1958. Bookchin and Gallop later identified HbA1c as a sugar-containing protein. But, most significantly, the clinical application of the HbA1c test was the work of the Iranian immunologist Samuel Rahbar.[13] While working at the University of Tehran a half-century ago, Dr. Rahbar noted that diabetics have increased levels of hemoglobin A1c. Suspecting, in view of its direct relation to blood sugar levels, that it may be of use in treating diabetes, he then extrapolated his metabolic data and determined it to be a major indicator of diabetes control.

The diabetic's goal is to keep his HbA1c below 7 percent. By checking a patient's HbA1c level, the doctor can detect the very presence of diabetes, or determine how well his patient is controlling his condition with medication, diet and exercise.

Although it is not standard practice to use HbA1c testing as a means of forecasting diabetes, recent scientific studies suggest that this test may be the best screening procedure for diabetes and pre-diabetes. Indeed, some researchers and clinicians feel that performing periodic HbA1c levels is the most accurate way of identifying future diatetics.[14] The normal HbA1c is less than 6 percent. An upward trend in the HbA1c toward 7 percent is an indication of an increasing risk of developing diabetes. If an upward trend is noted, early intervention can be instituted, and the future development of diabetes mellitus may, even in the presence of a genetic predisposition, be averted. Though not standard practice periodic HbA1c testing does make sense because the HbA1c value reflects an individual's average blood glucose level over a three month period; whereas the results of a fasting glucose test, even when repeated, hinges upon exactly when and what the individual has eaten on the day of the test, and when he last exercised.

The proposed diagnostic parameters are: HbA1c less than 6 percent

= normal, HbA1c of 6.1 percent–6.9 percent = pre-diabetic and HbA1c of 7 percent or greater = diabetic. People with kidney or liver disease, who are anemic or take vitamin C or E supplements, may have altered HbA1c results. Here in the U.S., the HbA1c is primarily used to assess the effectiveness of treatment (blood sugar control) of the already diagnosed type 2 diabetic. Curiously, in the U.S., it is rarely used as a diagnostic test. The reason: some insurance companies refuse to pay for it as a diagnostic test. Why should they, when in our market-medical economy, they can get away with a simple, less expensive fasting blood sugar test?

The Crux of the Matter — Why High Blood Sugar Is Harmful

Just as insulin is not needed to produce HbA1c, some normal body tissue cells do not require the presence of insulin to allow sugar to enter them. It is no coincidence that those tissues — the kidneys, blood vessels, lens of the eye, and nerves — are the very tissues at the root of all diabetic complications.[15] The cells of these tissues, it seems, have no natural barrier to keep sugar out; it seeps in directly, unimpeded. These cells become pickled with sugar, which, when metabolized, is changed into high-density sugar that draws in excess water by osmosis. This results in cellular damage. This process, unique to diabetics, is the basis for that most important imperative — in order to avoid complications, or at least minimize their effect, the diabetic patient must control his blood sugar (keep the HbA1c level down) and avoid dips and elevations.

The Importance of Insulin in Lipid Metabolism

Rarely, we come across a condition called *diabetic hyperlipemia*, literally — fat in the blood. In this condition, fat in the form of triglycerides (lipid) accumulates in the diabetic's blood to the extent that it can be easily observed with the naked eye. In a test tube, the fat appears as a thick white layer that rises to the top of the column of blood, like oil in a bottle of salad dressing. This condition, associated with accelerated atherosclerosis, results in heart attacks, strokes, and peripheral vascular disease and is caused by defective insulin metabolism. Diabetic hyperlipemia can be eliminated by the administration of insulin. This disease vividly demonstrates the importance of insulin, or the lack of it, in the lipid metabolism of the diabetic. The type 2 diabetic is plagued by inefficient lipid metabolism, and the result is high blood lipid levels (triglycerides), and elevated low density cholesterol.

Cholesterol, we shall see, is the major component of artery-obstructing plaque, and for Annie Walker, the underlying reason for a trip to the operating room.

Insulin as Medicine for the Non-diabetic

Many hormones can be manufactured by pharmaceutical companies and used to treat various diseases. Some examples: thyroid hormone for hypothyroidism, anabolic steroids, growth hormone, and testosterone for illicit use to enhance athletic performance, cortical-steroids to treat inflammatory diseases, and estrogen and progesterone for alleviation of menopausal symptoms, birth control, and maintenance of a youthful appearance. Estrogen is also used to create female breasts in males who change gender.

Recently, man-made insulin has been added to this list of general-purpose drugs. Critically ill patients, those in intensive care units throughout the world, are benefiting from the use of insulin as a medication. It has been recognized for some time now that the critically ill tend to have abnormally high blood sugar levels. This is the result of the increased production of hormones that kick in when the body is stressed: glucagon, growth hormone, and epinephrine. The critically ill are often treated with steroids, placed on high-calorie IV solutions, or given dialysis treatments, all therapies that boost blood sugar levels. Continuous high blood sugar levels, as we know, cause organ damage and increase the incidence and severity of infection in diabetics; so too with critically ill, non-diabetic patients.[16] Monitored insulin treatment in these non-diabetic, ICU patients improves metabolic function and thereby reduces the need for assisted mechanical ventilation. It lowers infection rates, decreases the need for dialysis treatments, and ultimately lowers mortality rates and shortens ICU stays.

You wouldn't think that cancer patients, non-diabetic cancer patients, who often lose weight and deal with the added stress of chemotherapy, have the highest blood glucose levels in the hospital, but they do.[17] It's not the cancer that raises their blood sugar levels it's the glucose-raising steroids and sugar-laden IV fluids they receive as part of their treatment. Studies have shown that if left untreated with insulin, these "temporary diabetics" have a higher mortality rate. The knowledgeable oncologist must treat the side effects of his treatment — temporary diabetes — as well as the cancer and, fortunately, most of them do.

Chapter 2

GENES, THE ENVIRONMENT, AND TYPE 2 DIABETES

Genetics plays a fundamental role in both types 1 and 2 diabetes, however the genetic defects are not the same. We have known for decades that type 1 diabetes is genetically based, because when it occurs in identical twins (who have the same genes), 50 percent to 60 percent of the time both twins inherit the condition. With fraternal twins (who have different genes), the incidence of both having the disease is only about 10 percent. A child with one parent affected with type 1 has a less than 10 percent chance of inheriting type 1 diabetes.

For the 90 percent of all diabetics with type 2, a genetic link has long been suspected. And if identical twins are an indicator, the link is even stronger than with type 1. If one twin has type 2, then there is a greater than 60 percent chance the other will have it as well. But the DNA details are only now becoming clear. The research arm of deCODE Genetics, a biotech company in Reykjavík, Iceland, has come up with some startling findings. We know from the company's work that 38 percent of the American population inherits the gene(s) for type 2 diabetes from one parent, giving those persons a 45 percent increased risk for type 2 diabetes.[1] An additional 7 percent of the population inherits the genes from both parents — making this group extremely likely to develop type 2 diabetes. On one point, all researchers agree: to express those genes, to become a type 2 diabetic, something must be added to the genetic mix — too many calories and too little exercise. These are the switches that activate the genes for type 2 diabetes. Even so, when you have no family history of type 2 diabetes, you still have an 11 percent chance of developing the disease by age 70, and sometimes genes play no role at all. The disease can occur as a side effect of medication or as a component of a seemingly unrelated disease.[2]

The Switch Works Anywhere in the World

Today, we think of the world's countries as underdeveloped, like parts of Africa and Asia; developing, like India and Pakistan; or developed, like the United States. Although type 2 diabetes can occur in any population, the disease is burgeoning in large, developed cities where folks find fast and processed foods affordable and convenient. So it is understandable that in more developed countries, the highest incidence of type 2 diabetes occurs in the lower income strata. Undeveloped countries, on the other hand, are almost free of the disease. Their inhabitants live off the land; they eat intrinsically healthy foods (or go hungry), and are physically active in harvesting those foods. The ancient genetic makeup of these people remains in sync with their more primitive lifestyle, food supply, and natural environment. Fast food restaurants and processed supermarket foods are not in their reach.

Those countries in between, developing countries such as India and Pakistan, are also plagued with an extremely high incidence of type 2 diabetes. In India's cities, however, there is a socioeconomic paradox — it is the rich who develop type 2 diabetes. Wealth provides the means to a valued social custom, the ability to buy and consume large quantities of pastries and sweets. Affording these foods connotes the cultural stamp of success, but at the same time provides a direct path to the development of type 2 diabetes.[3] Europe of the past couple of centuries had a similar situation, where consumption of a high protein diet with lots of meat, affordable only to the wealthy, caused rampant gout. In nineteenth century Europe, gout was considered a sign of affluence and social success; indeed, a status symbol. Similarly, in India today, a diagnosis of type 2 diabetes is an emblem of success (even if it's the physician who has the disease). Nearly 70 percent of India's population is rural, and yet these people are not exempt. Rural villagers have no fast food restaurants and they lack modern, energy-saving technology, but they've managed, by adopting the universal diet of fried, high-calorie foods and by living sedentary lives, to give India the highest prevalence of type 2 diabetes in the world.

Allopatric is the term biologists use to describe animal species that may once have coexisted, but have been separated by geologic events like the tectonic shifting of continents or rising sea levels, so their territories no longer overlap. Through random mutation over thousands of years, the genetic composition of these separated species changes to accommodate their unique environments. They evolve. In the extreme, separated species like African and Asian elephants or Bengal and Siberian tigers may evolve to the extent that even if reunited they can no longer interbreed. But unique geographic environments may produce less complex genetic variants that are still able to interbreed. We can include *Homo sapiens* in this group. Caucasian Europeans, Asiatic peoples, African Americans, Pacific Islanders, and too many other races to name can still produce offspring. Modern transportation technology has eliminated the geographic barriers that once kept them (and their genomes) apart. When divergent races comingle, they may pass on minute variations in their genetic makeup that can protect them from certain diseases, or make them soft targets for others. Studies by the NIH and the CDC and others have shown that Native Americans, Hispanic people, African Americans, Asians, and Pacific Islanders have brought with them the highest genetic predisposition, when the conditions are right, to develop type 2 diabetes.

Pre-diabetes — an Opportunity Often Missed

"What are my chances, Doc?" That's a line from an old movie. Actually, it's a question today's gravely ill rarely ask. Perceptive physicians can detect when patients fear answers and respect their need to be spared bad news. The healthy, on the other hand, do want to know their "chances," but not of dying. They want to know if they'll develop the same disease as a suffering sibling or parent.

That question is easily answered if the disease is type 1 diabetes. There is one chance in ten. For those with a family history of type 2 diabetes, the answer is: *that depends.* Many assume that if they carry the genes for a disease, they're destined to develop it, but this is not the case. Having the genes for type 2 diabetes is not a destiny; it's simply one of many risk factors. Geneticists, in most cases, can not determine if diabetes genes will express themselves, but now, at least, they can test for the tendency. In April 2007, deCODE Genetics, that same biotechnology company in Reykjavik, Iceland, through its commercial branch, DNA-Direct, was the first to offer these genetic tests.

When you seek a medical opinion regarding the odds of becoming diabetic, the doctor will usually order a fasting blood glucose test. If the laboratory returns a glucose value less than 100 mg percent, then for the present, the patient will be reassured. If the fasting blood glucose result is 126 mg percent or greater, then he is labeled diabetic. If the fasting blood glucose result falls between 101 and 126 mg percent, then he is considered to have impaired glucose tolerance — to be pre-diabetic. The label "pre-diabetic" is not to be taken lightly. Fortunately, it does not confirm a diabetic destiny. It means that if you reduce your risk by changing your lifestyle and eating habits, you still have an opportunity to avoid becoming a type 2 diabetic, or at least to delay the onset for many years. Pre-diabetes is a silent condition; there are no obvious signs or symptoms indicating its presence. Nearly 60 million Americans are pre-diabetic, according to the ADA. Most will develop type 2 diabetes and its inevitable complications within a decade. This is why the American Diabetes Association suggests that upon reaching age forty-five, we all have a fasting blood glucose test. If this seems like overkill, keep in mind that today, according to the National Institutes of Health, 12.9 percent of the U.S. population aged twenty or older has diabetes (with 7.7 percent diagnosed and 5.1 percent undiagnosed). And overall, 40 percent of the population has some type of high blood sugar condition.[4] It is no wonder that in the not-so-distant future a staggering one third of Americans will be overtly diabetic.

Overweight people who have a close relative with type 2 diabetes are considered high risk, and that risk is increased further in Native Americans, African Americans, Latinos, and Asian-Americans and Pacific Islanders. Overweight parents in this high-risk group would be smart to request periodic fasting glucose tests for their pre-teenagers. As high-risk ethnic groups intermingle, their diabetogenic genes are passed to their offspring.

Many chronic diseases incubate unnoticed. Type 2 diabetes is no exception. More often than not, pre-diabetes is diagnosed incidentally with a random blood chemistry test done for some other reason. If this is the case, the blood test should be repeated to confirm the diagnosis. Decades ago, when I was training, a test called the glucose tolerance test (GTT) was routinely used to diagnose diabetes. The glucose tolerance test, though rarely done now, is still considered slightly more sensitive than the usual diagnostic tests: fasting blood sugar, or repeated random blood sugar testing. It is considered the test of choice in the elderly, in whom the disease may be easily missed. (See Chapter 12.)

If your doctor says that you are pre-diabetic, then, in a sense, he is telling you that you are at a crossroad. If you continue straight through, that is, you remain overweight, enjoy a sedentary lifestyle, and eat what you like while ignoring the nutritional label on all packaged foods, then you've chosen the wrong route. If you make a turn, lose weight, start exercising, and follow your physician's advice regarding blood sugar, blood pressure, cholesterol, and triglyceride control with the proper medications, then you are likely to avoid or delay becoming a type 2 diabetic. Most important, you will delay dealing with the inevitable complications.

It is true that the diagnostic criteria, hence the labels "pre-diabetic" and "diabetic," are based solely on your blood sugar level. Historically, we think of diabetes as a sugar problem in overweight people, but 20 percent of type 2 diabetics are not overweight. In fact, high blood sugars do not cause most of the blood vessel-based complications of type 2 diabetes. These are the result of genetically associated defects in cholesterol and lipid metabolism as well as untreated high blood pressure — and being overweight is not a prerequisite; it is simply another risk factor.

Extensive research over many years has shown that treating high blood sugar alone is not sufficient to prevent diabetic complications. Proper medications must be prescribed to control blood pressure, cholesterol and lipids. With this in mind, the American Diabetes Association has set guidelines for doctors and patients to follow to control cholesterol and lipids, and for blood pressure management. Unfortunately, physicians who do not specialize in the treatment of diabetes often don't follow these clinical guidelines.[5]

Lifestyles and Disease in the Animal Kingdom

The longest-lived vertebrate in the United States is the box turtle — at 125 years.[6] Yes, turtles are vertebrates; their spines are fused to the inner surface of their shell. The box turtle has specific nutritional requirements, and no choice but to stick to them. This tortoise lives slowly and has a metabolism to match. It evolved that way to assure survival during long intervals without food and to tolerate adverse weather conditions. When food is available — berries, earthworms, fallen apples — the tortoise will gorge itself. When food is scarce, it will retire from sight and enter a hibernation-like state. It estivates. The dietary swings have no obvious ill effect.

The giant tortoises of the Galapagos Islands serve as a good example of the slow end of an adjustable metabolism, one that came in handy not only for them, but for the whaling men of the 1820's. In his book, *In the Heart of the Sea,* Nathaniel Philbrick tells the true version of the tragedy of the Essex, the whaleship and crew that inspired the epic Moby Dick. In the 1800's, whaleships spent years on the open sea before returning to their home ports. After setting out from Nantucket, the Essex sailed to the Galapagos to not only hunt sperm whales, but to provision-up. There they collected scores of giant, hundred-pound, tortoises and stacked them live upside down in the hold or let them walk the deck. Fresh food was a luxury. "One of the reasons the tortoises were so valued by the whalemen was because they could live for more than a year without food or water. Not only was the tortoise's meat still plump and tasty, but it also yielded eight to ten pounds of fat."[7]

At the other end of the spectrum — the fast end — is the hummingbird. Each day it sucks in sugary nectar equaling twice its body weight. One half of that fluid is pure sugar. This would be the equivalent of a 150-pound man eating 150 pounds of sugar each day. The hummingbird supplements its diet with protein in the form of fruit flies and small flying insects. Some species of hummingbirds have wings that beat at an invisible 300 times per second. And some of these delicate birds, including the tiny rubythroat, the only hummingbird east of the Mississippi, migrate over 1,000 miles each winter to the Gulf of Mexico.[8] This frenetic activity dissipates the huge sugar load and maintains their lean body habitus. When food can't be found, or the weather is cold, the hummingbird finds a sheltered perch and, like the tortoise, goes into a torpid state; its heart rate and metabolism slow down to conserve energy.

The box turtle and the hummingbird are equipped with a metabolism precisely set to mesh with its changing environment. They, like all creatures (except humans), have no choice but to live in a manner that insures their survival. Their diet and energy expenditure are genetically hardwired to harmonize with their surroundings. Whether you interpret this natural imperative as Darwinian adaptation and natural selection or as God's creation makes no difference. The inability of these creatures to choose a lifestyle — or possibly make a fatal decision — assures their individual wellbeing as well as their survival as a species.

We humans (*Homo sapiens,* smart man) are the fragile ones. For us, missing lunch is a hardship. We are no longer equipped with the protective mechanisms of so-called lower life forms. Their metabolic parameters, exercise requirements, and diets are inborn, instinctively set in a narrow range. Ours are not. Our limits have been lifted, manipulated by large brains that let us make choices and set our own lifestyle. Consequently, what we eat and how we expend energy are conscious choices. We have a metabolic need to eat regularly, but unfortunately we lack the impulse control and the environmental constraints needed to eat wisely. Moreover, the obligation of healthful physical activity has been lifted, replaced by the many energy-saving devices of our industrialized world.

The once lean-and-mean poor have morphed into chubby, complacent consumers of fast food. The minimum wage in the United States, though it varies from state to state, remains embarrassingly low, so eating healthy is often not an option for the working poor. Anyone can succumb to the bombardment of fast food advertising, but those of us with the genes for type 2 diabetes or the metabolism of a tortoise lack the ability to properly utilize these carbohydrate rich, excessively fatty, calorie-laden, foods. It is no wonder that with the globalization of the American diet, especially those aspects catering to the indiscreet consumer and the poor, we are experiencing an exponential rise, worldwide, in the incidence of type 2 diabetes.

Our physical activity requirements have been reduced by industrialization. We don't walk; we ride. We don't farm; we shop. We do what we can to eliminate the "burden" of physical activity. Yet, surprisingly, we're sleep deprived. We watch television and surf the net. We spend our time in the bus, train, or car commuting to and from work — work that's likely more cognitive than physical. A study done at Yale University School of Medicine has identified sleep duration as a risk factor for the development of type 2 diabetes. Researchers there noted that Americans sleep an average of 6.8 hours per night, whereas one hundred years ago, we slept 8.3 hours per night. Over a fifteen-year period they documented the metabolic alterations associated with sleep deprivation. They noted a detrimental effect on insulin resistance (the key to sugar metabolism). The researchers concluded that "sleep curtailment may predispose individuals to overt clinical diabetes." But it works both ways; too much sleep has been studied as well, and it too is considered a risk factor.[9]

A Natural Experiment in Lifestyles

Without a doubt, the most blatant example of lifestyle change leading to type 2 diabetes involves the Tohono O'odham Indians of Pima

County, Arizona. This Native American tribe, part of the Pima Indian Nation, is studied intensively by diabetes researchers. Unwittingly, its members have made themselves the principal participants in an unplanned natural experiment. Three out of four Tohono O'odham Indians, that's 75 percent, have diabetes mellitus. Ninety five percent are afflicted with type 2. Pima County, Arizona, is the epicenter of diabetes mellitus in the United States. Spanish Harlem in New York City ranks a close second.[10] But as far as entire countries are concerned, India boasts the highest prevalence.[11]

For thousands of years, the lifestyles of Native Americans, Asians, Hispanics, African Americans and Caucasians were restricted by their natural surroundings. They, like all other creatures, were protected by a pristine environment. They were free from obesity, type 2 diabetes, and other manmade diseases. Gradually, assimilation into the post industrial world changed their lifestyles. Their new, unnatural, artificial environment enabled them to activate their sleeping genes for type 2 diabetes and exposed them to a host of additional maladies. For thousands of years the Tohono O'odham Indians of Pima County were able to subsist, even thrive, in the arid Arizona desert.[12] They ate what they grew, mainly squash, corn, and beans. In the remote desert, they hunted small game and foraged for cactus fruit and cactus pads. They were slender and fit; the human version of the box turtle. Their genetic makeup allowed them to thrive in their natural surroundings. As cities sprung up around them, they remained tightly knit, even as the tribe adopted the ways of the modern world. They lost their farming and gathering skills and replaced them with new ones: shopping for food bargains and consuming processed foods with high sugar and saturated fat contents. (A cheeseburger and fries for a dollar beats scouring the desert for cactus pads, and it's cheaper than cooking at home.) Ironically, the American Indian had become "Americanized." The Arizona Pima Indians are unwitting victims of a global catastrophe. They've adopted the now omnipresent diet of the masses, fast foods. The availability of cheap but nutritionally disastrous foods coupled with a sedentary lifestyle has awakened the dormant genes for type 2 diabetes and, for them, caused a health catastrophe replete with the distinct possibilities of amputations, blindness, kidney failure, and heart disease.

But luckily for the researchers, centuries ago a group of Tohono O'odham Pima Indians left Arizona. They split from the main tribe and migrated hundreds of miles, settling in a remote, almost inaccessible part of the Mexican Sierra Nevada Mountains. In scientific terms, they had become a control group — an accidental control group. Diabetes researchers from multiple collaborating scientific centers seized the rare opportunity to study and compare the two groups. Unlike the modern Pima Indians of Arizona, the primitive Mexican Pimas continue to live in isolation. Only occasional farmers and ranchers share the isolated land of the Mexican Pimas. Having once been a part of a single large Pima Indian Nation, the Mexican Pimas have retained the common language, traditions and customs of the Pimas of Arizona, and, most significant — the two groups share the same basic genetic makeup. Today, their lifestyles alone set them apart. The Arizona Pimas have adopted our typical industrialized American lifestyle; the Mexican Pimas live off the land, in isolation.

The researchers learned, or perhaps simply confirmed, that the leaner, more physically active Mexican Pima Indians have a significantly lower incidence of type 2 diabetes.[13] The incidence of type 2 diabetes in Mexican Pima men is six times lower than in their urbanized counterparts in Arizona. And amongst women, the incidence of type 2 diabetes is 5.5 times lower than in the Arizona Pima females. A natural experiment has provided proof that lifestyle — eating habits and exercise — is a stronger influence than simple genetic makeup in the development of type 2 diabetes.

One way to explain the Arizona Pimas' fate is through *epigenetics*. Most of us remember Gregor Mendel, the Austrian monk who studied the inheritance patterns of common garden peas — 28,000 of them. Through his observations of pea plants' color, stem length, seed size, etc., he came up with the laws of genetics. He published his work in the 1860s, but his data went unnoticed by the scientific community. Even Darwin failed to see the vital connection with his theory of natural selection. Mendel joined many great scientists whose work was recognized only after they'd died. Now high-school texts refer to him as the Father of Genetics.

Mendel's inheritance hypothesis was relatively simple. Of necessity, it was hatched purely from observation and mathematics-based theory, as the study of DNA, chromosome structure, and biogenetics were yet to come. With a keen eye and careful cross-breeding (he pollinated the 28,000 plants himself), Mendel was able to accurately predict the physical appearance of his pea plants. He coined the terms *dominant* and *recessive* traits, but instead of "genes," he used the terms "units" and "factors." The word gene was first used a half century later in 1909, when Mendel's work was rediscovered by the Danish botanist Wilhelm Johannsen. Only then was Mendel's accomplishment recognized and finally taken seriously.

It wasn't until 1942 that the term *epigenetics* came into use. This word, first used by the British embryologist Conrad Hal Waddington (1905–1975), describes how a gene's expression (its phenotype) can be altered by the environment. This is a key concept in the understanding of type 2 diabetes. To understand the meaning of epigenetics, consider a clutch of turtle eggs. When incubated in warmth, it will hatch out all female turtles. If incubated below a certain temperature (in a cool environment), all the eggs will hatch out males. Or consider the color of hydrangeas, which bloom blue if grown in acid soil, but pink if grown in an alkaline garden. Waddington, like many great scientists, was a thinker; his data derived from observation, his laboratory was his brain, for in 1942 the physical appearance and function of genes had not yet been defined. That, the secret of life, the structure of DNA, was only brought to light in 1953 by James Watson and Francis Crick. Today, we realize that Mendel's units of inheritance, genes (or factors as he called them), can be coaxed into altering their expression, and moreover, biochemists have accurately determined the chemical adjustments responsible for tweaking them to do so. Key to understanding the diabetes "epidemic" is knowing that these altered genes — "environmentally influenced genes" (or man-made alterations, for that matter) — may be passed from generation to generation. This has great significance when considering the plight of the Tohono Indians and helps to explain the rapid rise, worldwide, of type 2 diabetes and obesity. Perhaps you're old enough to remember reading about the nineteenth-century French scientist Jean-Baptiste Lamarck. We laughed up our sleeves when, in high school, we learned he'd suggested that acquired traits could be passed from generation to generation. Well, he was right — for the wrong reasons, but he was right.*

Now, in the twenty-first century, science has progressed from rudimentary studies of pea plants in Mendel's monastery gardens to the international achievement of mapping the human genome. The biggest scientific project in history, mapping the human genome, was begun in 1991. It involves hundreds of scientists from the U.S., China, France, Germany, Japan, and Great Britain and has cost about $3 billion. The last of

---

*Lamarck believed that an animal's altered lifestyle might trigger a change in its anatomy which could then be passed to subsequent generations. For example, he believed that giraffes who stretched to feed on higher leaves would lengthen their necks and those long necks would then be passed directly to the next generation. In fact, he was proposing, decades before the concept of genetics was defined, that environment influences an organism's anatomic (and necessarily its metabolic) characteristics and that those peculiarities could then be passed down through generations.

our 46 chromosomes was mapped in 2006. Such a colossal endeavor had to wait for the digital age in order to splice together the findings of so many geneticists.

Motivated by the colossal global burden of type 2 diabetes, scientists have tapped into this treasure trove to determine the effect of a person's genome on the probability of becoming diabetic. There are some 25,000 genes in human DNA; so far, only about a dozen and a half have been implicated as significant-risk genes for the development of type 2 diabetes. "What," these scientists asked, "would most accurately predict one's chances of developing the disease?" Would it be a genotypic score (the number of risk genes a person carries), or simply adding up an individual's known environmental risk factors? Two major, independent retrospective studies were done, one in Europe, and the other in the U.S. Combined, the studies had 21,208 participants. In the U.S. study, 2,770 people were followed, some for over twenty-three years. In the European study, 16,106 subjects were followed for up to twenty-eight years. The studies compared a total of 21 risk genes to easily-identified risk factors such as family history, body weight, high blood pressure, triglyceride levels, etc. The two studies reached the same conclusion: knowing an individual's genetic makeup helps little, if at all, to help predict his chances of becoming a type 2 diabetic.[11] Bottom line — genes are important, but how you live, what you eat and how you interact with your environment are, for the most part, what determine if you will become a type 2 diabetic.[14]

The Thrifty Gene Theory: A Likely Explanation of Why We Americans Are Becoming Fat and Diabetic

One man, a geneticist, saw it coming. On a genetic level, the differences between the lean, fit Tohono Indians of Mexico and the chubby, complacent diabetic Tohono Indians of Arizona can be explained, in part, by the "thrifty gene theory" of James V. Neel. Neel was a scientist who taught at the University of Michigan. Geneticists (not high school science books) refer to him as the Father of Human Genetics. In the 1960s, Neel theorized that certain populations of people are protected, in much the same way as the tortoise and the hummingbird, by their unique genetic makeup. He postulated that many distinct populations, including Native Americans, Pacific Islanders, Australian aborigines, and various nomadic peoples have, as part of their ancient gene pool, a "thrifty gene" which enables them to survive in times of famine and allows them to gorge themselves in times of plenty. This gene gave its possessors the ability to survive in rough times — when crop harvests were poor, foraging was unproductive, and hunting was futile — and it permitted them to fatten up without consequence in times of plenty.

These distinct populations evolved unique genomes, perfect fits to ensure not only their survival, but their ability to thrive in their particular environments. Their metabolisms were fine tuned over thousands of years to function with maximal efficiency on the fuel provided by their environment, and the octane of that fuel was designed to meet their specific energy needs. Just as the beaks and bodies of Darwin's Galapagos's finches enabled them to flourish on the native seeds of their unique island habitats, the physical and metabolic needs of Pacific Islanders, nomadic peoples, and Native Americans allowed them to thrive in their natural habitats. But Darwin's finches had small brains. If a storm took them to an inhospitable island where they were unable to adjust, they would likely die or return from whence they came. But we are *Homo sapiens—smart* man; when we change environments or create industrialized ecosystems, we make do, we don't die. We adapt, but our invisible metabolic needs are not really met, so we don't thrive. We develop type 2 diabetes.

As civilizations progress, lifestyles are altered. Societal changes occur quickly, sometimes within a few years. On the other hand, our genetic makeup, the blueprint for bodily function, remains essentially stable for thousands, or more likely millions of years. In civilized societies, food is plentiful, cyclic famines disappear and the need to expend energy on hunting, foraging, and planting is eliminated. The thrifty gene is no longer needed; it becomes a disadvantage. For the Tohono Indians of Pima County, Arizona, and for us, too, this once advantageous thrifty gene now functions only to allow obesity, to morph its holder from fit to fat and diabetic. Obesity causes insulin resistance (the inability of insulin to carry sugar into the cells). When you turn up the dial on insulin resistance, you tune in type 2 diabetes. However, for the isolated, self-sufficient, fast food–deprived Tohono Indians of Mexico, the thrifty gene is still an asset.

During and before the Civil War, life expectancy in the United States was less than 50 years. People often died from conditions that are easily cured today — ruptured appendices, complicated childbirths, and pneumonia, to name a few. Type 1 diabetes, when it appeared, was quickly fatal (prior to 1921, with the isolation of insulin by Banting and Best), and very few people lived long enough to develop type 2 diabetes. If they survived beyond 50, chances are they were thin and more likely malnourished than obese. Today, moderate longevity and obesity, coupled with genetic potential, are the stepping stones to type 2 diabetes. It is not unusual these days to see patients who have had both their appendix and their gallbladder removed. They may be cancer survivors, have a coronary artery stent or two, and may take a variety of medications, all of which have lengthened their lives and, in the process, given them the dubious opportunity to develop type 2 diabetes.

Types 1 and 2 diabetes are, at once, similar and separate diseases. With the exception of those with latent autoimmune diabetes in the adult (LADA), the onset of type 1 diabetes occurs in youth, sometimes as early as four or five years of age, sometimes as late as 25 or 28. Type 1 diabetes was formerly called *juvenile diabetes*, however, with the recently described LADA variation of type 1 diabetes, and the increasingly earlier in life onset of type 2 diabetes, the term *juvenile diabetes* is no longer appropriate. Yet from a surgical point of view, the variety of complications resulting from types 1 and 2 are indistinguishable.

During my 35 years as a surgeon, I have noticed a blurring of the clinical line between type 1 and 2 diabetics. Type 2 diabetes is appearing earlier in life and this provides more time for the development of complications. Because of this, children and young adults with type 2 diabetes often deal with its complications while in the prime of life. The most frequent complication is neuropathy, nerve damage which takes many forms but is most often manifested as a loss of pain sensation in the feet. Other complications — kidney failure, arterial disease, heart disease or blindness — may appear in any order, in any given patient. But bear in mind, for some the disease is imperceptible, hidden in a blood test yet to be taken. Unfortunately for them, the complications may appear even before the diagnosis is exposed.

Type 1 diabetics rely on insulin injections to control their blood sugar. With no insulin of their own, they have no choice. Typically, from the start, type 1s are prone to wide swings in their blood sugar levels. These swings cause unpleasant side effects: nausea, vomiting, sweating, loss of concentration — jarring reminders that reinforce the necessity of blood sugar control. Not to do so could easily be fatal. On the other hand, typical type 2 diabetics do not experience these dramatic symptomatic episodes until late in their disease when they, too, may become insulin dependent. When first diagnosed, type 2s often consider their disease as simply "a sugar problem." All the while, as their brains are minimizing their condition, the drip, drip, drip of silent disease is causing their bodies to undergo the pathologic metamorphosis that leads to life-altering blood vessel, nerve and organ damage.

Denial is easy for the type 2 diabetic, especially early on when symptoms are absent and the physician has nothing but a blood test to treat. So it is no surprise that type 1 diabetics are more aware of self-preservation and better at caring for their disease. They are forced to learn, from an early age, a most important lesson — keeping their blood sugar normal and avoiding dips and elevations is, in no uncertain terms, the best way to avoid complications or at least minimize their effect.

Of necessity, type 1 diabetics, who are often children, have built-in advocates, their parents. An advocate, someone who watches over your situation, is particularly important in today's atmosphere of fragmented medical care. Most diabetics, for several reasons, would benefit from an advocate on an everyday basis. One reason is that the diabetic's decision making process may be impaired by swings in his blood sugar. Another is that here in the United States, medical care has changed from a one-on-one doctor/patient relationship to an impersonal healthcare industry which makes the patient a consumer of often disjointed and complex services and technology. Ideally, every diabetic would benefit from someone, other than just his doctor, to watch over him. Someone to remind him of his ABCs: that careful control of his blood sugar–A1c, Blood pressure, and Cholesterol medications is the most effective way to decrease or delay the occurrence of diabetic complications. It is unfortunate, however, that even the most fastidious diabetic, one who takes his condition seriously and cares for it implicitly, can still develop the life-altering surgical complications of diabetes.

Who's to Blame for This Scourge?

Type 2 diabetes has been labeled a "lifestyle disease," and so it would seem that the diabetic may harbor some guilt, and that those around him might even assign blame. After all, syphilis is a lifestyle disease and so is alcoholic cirrhosis of the liver. But, these days, in view of our complex, industrialized societies, choosing a lifestyle is not a simple matter. We live in a diabetogenic world. The lifestyle risks are built in. They greet us at every turn: in our restaurants, our supermarkets, our cars and airplanes, in our easy chairs, and, of course, they lurk in our jeans.... my mistake — our genes.

Physicians are hesitant to cast blame. But let's face it; type 2 diabetes is not the result of some communicable bacterium or mosquito-borne virus. It hardly existed before the Civil War. I'm not an epidemiologist; I don't trace the origins of disease, but looking back, it's obvious. If someone is responsible for this forest fire, it's Eli Whitney. He lit the match. Yes, Eli Whitney, the same guy responsible for the Civil War.

"How so?" you ask. Because in 1793, the Yankee Eli Whitney invented the cotton gin. This simple time- and energy-saving piece of machinery marked the start of the industrial revolution. Textile mills sprung up in the North and boosted the economy; meanwhile, wealthy Southerners depended on four million slaves to harvest their lucrative cotton crop for export throughout the world. By 1860 cotton was our biggest export, totaling $191million in revenue.[15] The United States became ideologically divided. Northerners, financially independent and with no need for slaves, were able to see the immoral implications of the system. Southerners, morally blindfolded by their newfound wealth from cotton exports, depended on slavery. With slavery the crucial issue, the Civil War erupted.

As for Eli's role in the diabetes epidemic, his invention, the cotton gin, launched the industrial revolution. Industrialization is a one-way street with no speed limit. With the industrialization of our food supply and our transportation systems, our lifestyles were permanently transformed — the scene was set for our obesity and diabetes epidemics.

We did not consciously reconstruct our environment, hence our lifestyles, to be conducive to diabetes, but if someone is to blame — I'll point my finger at Eli Whitney.

Chapter 3

WHY OBESITY LEADS TO TYPE 2 DIABETES

Obesity is the emblem of the type 2 diabetic and a major risk factor—yet it is not a prerequisite. Many type 2 diabetics, over 20 percent, are not overweight. Obese people have excess or greatly enlarged fat cells. In lay terms, the words obese, fat, overweight, chubby, etc. are simply subjective descriptions. According to the scientific community, obesity is not merely a body habitus; it is a condition likely to result in disease. In addition to diabetes, obesity—a high body mass index (BMI), the scientific measure of obesity—often leads to hypertension, elevated LDL (bad cholesterol), decreased HDL (good cholesterol), high triglyceride levels in the blood, coronary artery disease, stroke, gallstones, arthritis, sleep apnea, and uterine, breast and colon cancer. There are those who will argue that physically fit overweight people are as healthy as normal-weight folks who are not fit. Scientists seesaw on this subject, but there is no question — regular exercise curbs the development of type 2 diabetes and, for those already afflicted, eases control. And, for the overweight individual the single most effective method of avoiding type 2 diabetes is sustained weight reduction.

The BMI is measured by employing a standard mathematical formula calculated from a person's height, weight and a conversion factor. This formula is used by the Centers for Disease Control and Prevention (CDC) to scientifically define obesity. The BMI is more than a scientific measure of obesity; it is a very accurate predictor of your chances of developing type 2 diabetes. In order to calculate your BMI using pounds and inches the formula is: your weight divided by your height in inches squared, times 703 (the conversion factor). So, for a 150-pound man whose height is 65 inches, the calculation of the BMI would be as follows: 150 / 65² × 703 = 24.96. Under the metric system, the formula for a person whose weight is 68 kg. and whose height is 165 cm. (1.65 m), the calculation is 68 / 1.65² × 703 = 24.96.

For adults over 20 years of age, regardless of sex, your BMI determines whether or not you are obese. Simply stated, the doctor can say, "You're fat, and I can prove it!" In many cases, however, he can not distinguish whether your obesity stems from a genetic propensity or simply from overeating. But who, you may wonder, had the audacity to set the standard, and when was it done? Good question. The first mathematical formulas to define obesity were worked out in the 1870s by a French surgeon, Dr. P.P. Broca. In the 1970s the formula was modified for use by insurance companies to predict life expectancy, and by pharmaceutical companies to calculate dosage. Medical science popularized the formula as it became more apparent that obesity and ill health go hand in hand. The designation of obesity — a BMI score of 30 or higher — was, appropriately, set in the 1970s, just at the start of the fast food/obesity revolution.

For children the BMI is age- and sex-specific, so the calculation is altered, but if the child's BMI is above the 95th percentile (using height and weight data from the 1970s) he is considered obese. The normal BMI for any adult male or female is 18.5 to 24.9. Overweight is defined as 25 to 29.9 and obese is defined as having a BMI score above 30. You can check your BMI on the Web (Google BMI) and plug your height and weight into the provided formula to calculate your own.

Presently, according to the scientific community's definition, abnormal lipid metabolism takes place when an individual ingests excess calories. It does not matter whether those calories come from carbohydrate, fat or protein. Incidentally, animal or vegetable fats contain twice the number of calories (8.8 cal.), gram for gram, as carbohydrate (3.9 cal.) or protein (3.9 cal.). Alcohol has 7 calories/gram. (Animal fat, though, is bad for you, while most vegetable fat is not.) Those calories which are not used as fuel for your body's normal metabolism or for physical exercise are stored as fat, adipose tissue. Consider this; it takes one hour of moderately fast walking to burn off the 250 calories provided by one cupcake. If, instead of exercising after you eat, you take a nap (the sumo wrestler's trick for gaining weight), that cupcake's calories turn into fat.

The body's normal anatomical fat stores (the subcutaneous tissue, the fatty tissues around your internal organs, and the omental apron, your internal abdominal fat pad) cannot safely pack in excess fat molecules. The result is an abnormal development of fat cells in and around organs where fat is not usually found. This is called ectopic fat. Fat cells may appear in non-adipose tissues: primarily the liver, skeletal muscle, around intra-abdominal organs (visceral fat), and among the pancreatic beta cells. Every surgeon has observed that normal-weight women have more subcutaneous fat and normal-weight men have more visceral fat. During surgery on all obese patients, we encounter abundant visceral fat and note that the liver's appearance is altered. Fat cells invading liver tissue give the organ a yellowish tint and the liver's edges become round and plump instead of knife-sharp.

Fat cells accumulating in or around organs where fat is not usually found is called ectopic fat; within the abdomen it's called visceral fat.[1] These excessive fat deposits are particularly dangerous because they generate toxins called *cytokines*. Cytokines cause insulin resistance and the eventual deterioration of beta cell function. So excess body fat actually functions like a giant, out of control endocrine gland which, through cytokine production, causes insulin resistance; the metabolic defect responsible for type 2 diabetes. This is how obesity leads to high blood sugars and type 2 diabetes.[2]

But there is an important distinction to be made between visceral fat and subcutaneous fat—a distinction, that is, between being chubby and possessing a pot belly. Waist size matters[3] for two reasons: because that extra intra-abdominal or visceral fat—to a far greater extent than subcutaneous fat—secretes those cytokines and hormones which result in insulin resistance, the pivotal cause of type 2 diabetes, and because cytokines in the blood are "markers of systemic inflammation," which, we shall see, increase the risk for cardiovascular disease.[4]

Case Two: The Diabetic Foot

My office is on the first floor of a high-rise building. No steps. It's easier for the amputees, folks with walkers, wheelchairs, or the just plain lame. My desk chair faces the window beside the walkway leading to the office door. I keep the blinds up so I can see my unsuspecting charges approach. Do they smoke? Limp? Require assistance? I don't see them all, but occasionally I spot a piece of the puzzle that explains my patient's plight. Most surgeons have office hours only half a day, once or twice a week. The rest of the time we're in the hospital, usually in the O.R. My office days are

3. Why Obesity Leads to Type 2 Diabetes

Monday afternoons and Thursday mornings. I see new patients and post-ops, and I usually squeeze in one or two emergency consultations.

One Monday afternoon I observed my first patient, a well-insulated, middle-aged woman, as she limped from her car up the walkway to the office door. After twenty feet or so she'd stop and rest, then walk again. She was favoring her right foot; protecting the left.

Two chubby boys trailed behind her. The two kids, it turns out, were the grandchildren. One was eight, the other ten. Mom, having found a parking space, was last in line. As the four ambled up the walk, a vision of ducklings flashed through my brain. Grandma entered first. She stopped at the reception window. Gail, my nurse, noted her insurance information, and then took her and her daughter to my examining room. The two boys sat quietly in the waiting room, their heads down, thumbing their video games and sharing a bag of Fritos. Gail escorted Grandma to a sturdy chair. She sat. Mom entered, glanced at the stool, the only other place to sit, and remained standing.

Grandma's name was Louise. She'd been a type 2 diabetic for 22 years. Over that time she had progressed from diet control to pills to insulin. She had had no serious diabetes-related problems, she told me, until the previous Thursday, when she opened her freezer door to retrieve a lasagna. As she reached up to slide it out she dislodged a frozen chicken; it tumbled out and smashed her right big toe. By Friday, the nail was black. By Sunday it was raised off its bed, and by the time I saw her, only four days later, the entire toe was red and swollen. Yellow pus oozed from under that barely attached nail.

We went through the details of her history: diabetes for 22 years, on insulin. Tests her blood sugar before breakfast, supper and at bedtime. She kept a log book as all insulin dependent diabetics should. Each page contained seven days of data: the date, blood sugar readings at breakfast, lunch, dinner, and bedtime, why and which medications she took, and "comments." She paged through it, then looked up, and, as if to say, "It wasn't my fault," pointed to Thursday's entry. It read: "Dropped chicken on right big toe." She'd noted her elevated blood sugars over the past three days, and the increased insulin dose needed to cover them. As she slipped the log book back into her purse a pack of Marlboros peeked out. She volunteered, "I only smoke two or three a day."

Her daughter tossed her head back and rolled her eyes; she wanted to speak, but managed for a moment to keep quiet. Then she mumbled, "She drinks, too."

"How much?" I asked, pondering the surprising benefits of moderate alcohol consumption on diabetics.

"One drink after dinner. That's all," Louise admitted.

"That's not a problem," I told her, "as long as you keep it to one drink; and make sure you've eaten first. Diabetics who drink on an empty stomach can get a sudden drop in blood sugar and pass out." (Type 2 diabetics actually benefit from light to moderate alcohol consumption. Alcohol is caloric, but in the diabetic, through its actions on the liver, it acts like a potent blood sugar-lowering drug. Moreover, taken in moderation, it lowers blood lipid levels, decreases insulin resistance, and acts as an anti-inflammatory agent.)[5] I asked Louise about her family. She told me her father had passed away thirty years ago. He was not a diabetic. Then the daughter revealed that she had recently been diagnosed with pre-diabetes. She was trying to keep it from progressing by watching her diet. I knew that wasn't enough. I asked about the boys. The women gave me a quizzical look. "Oh, no, they're only eight and ten," they said as one.

"Have they been tested?" I asked.

"No."

"Have them tested," I said. "Even at eight and ten, if the conditions are right, we're seeing type 2 diabetes." They nodded.

Louise eased off her right shoe using her left foot and the left shoe using her right. She couldn't reach her feet. Gail gave her a gown. I left the room. When I returned, Gail, the daughter and I hoisted Grandma onto the examining table. I felt her pulses. They were bounding in both groins. The pulse behind the right knee (the popliteal pulse) was normal, but the pulse behind the left knee was absent. I placed my finger tips on the posterior tibial and then dorsalis pedis arteries in each foot. On the right, the pulses were good. I felt nothing, however, on the left. Now the limp made sense; it had nothing to do with the chicken.

I listened to her neck for evidence of carotid artery stenosis (narrowing). There was no whistling sound, no bruit. I examined her belly knowing that even if she had an aortic aneurysm, her bulk would hide it from me. I told her that despite her diabetes, the circulation in her right foot was quite good. And in order to reassure her, I placed my Doppler probe over the dorsalis pedis artery on the top of her foot so she could hear the loud, crisp flow. Then, on the left, we heard the faint whisper of obstructed blood flow. She was fortunate, I told her, that the chicken chose her good foot. Normal blood flow lets you walk without pain and, for Louise, would be the key to healing. Had it landed on the left, she'd be facing a difficult time.

I explained that in order to properly drain her infection, the toenail had to be removed. I knew that with the bounding pulses in her right foot, and in the absence of a bone infection (osteomyelitis), proper wound care and antibiotics would result in prompt healing. Osteomyelitis takes almost 2 weeks to show up on an X-ray. Her problem was less than a week old, so I didn't order one. It was too early, too, for an MRI, the best test to detect osteomyelitis.

Without giving her time to think, I pulled on some sterile gloves, swabbed the toe with antiseptic, gripped the nail tightly with a clamp, and yanked it off. I used no local anesthetic. I knew it wouldn't hurt; the nail was hardly attached and her diabetes left her neuropathic — she no longer felt pain in her feet. It didn't bleed. I took a culture and handed the swab to Gail. With the toenail gone and the abscess drained, the strong pulses in that foot set the stage for healing. I showed her how to change the bandage. "Change it four times a day," I told her.

I gave her no Rx for antibiotics — better to wait for the culture report. It would take a day or two, but ensure she got the specific antibiotic designed to kill the bacterium causing her infection. No shotgun therapy here. I explained how to elevate the foot of her bed and told her I'd see her in a week; we'd talk about the other leg then. I returned to my office. She dressed, gathered her daughter and the boys and left. I watched through the window as they walked to their car — single file!

Is Obesity Genetic?

Are there genetic variations that affect your metabolism? And, if there are, can they be passed from generation to generation? For decades, scientists have used laboratory rats to study these questions. In the 1960s, while working at the laboratory of comparative anatomy in Massachusetts, Drs. Theodore and Lois Zucker were able to breed a strain of rats which are extremely large and very fat. They are so obese they can't curl up in a ball to sleep. They rest on their backs, feet in the air. They are two and a half times the weight and size of normal laboratory rats. These giant genetic variants are called Zucker fatty rats.

In their efforts to study the genetics of obesity, over a period of twenty-five years, researchers subjected this strain of obese rats to repeated inbreeding. Over time their genetic makeup was channeled into yet a new strain — jumbo rats. Each jumbo rat carries a pair of mutant (fa) genes;

one from the father, the buck, and one from the mother, the doe. These are the genes for obesity. If jumbo rats are fed a normal diet, they remain large, but not fat. But give them unlimited food, they'll eat it non-stop and become obese. So, not surprisingly, when these super sized rats approach rat middle age, they develop type 2 diabetes.[6] However, if their diet is carefully restricted with regard to quantity, carbohydrate, and fat intake, and if they are forced to exercise regularly, that is, placed on an exercise wheel, then they remain oversized, but avoid becoming type 2 diabetics. They are the laboratory equivalent of the human type 2 diabetic, complete with all the complications from neuropathy to kidney failure.

This new strain is called the Zucker diabetic fatty rats. The Zuckers, through their genetic research, isolated a specific gene mutation (fa) on chromosome 5. This deranged or mutated gene is responsible in part, for the rat's obesity. The mutated gene (fa) causes two major alterations in the jumbo rat's biochemistry: insulin resistance, and an inability of the pancreatic beta cells to compensate by increasing insulin production. Normal-sized, or wild-type laboratory rats, on the other hand have unimpaired insulin metabolism They are not diabetic because that particular gene is not mutated. Rather than (fa), they carry the normal gene (Fa) on chromosome 5. The specific genetic pathways may differ slightly in humans and rats, but the result is the same — type 2 diabetes.

Fat is not merely insulation — fat functions. Body fat, you see, secretes hormones. One's body fat cells (the lipocytes) act in concert, as if they are a giant endocrine gland. One such hormone, leptin, functions in part to control body weight. It is part of the body's natural defense against obesity. If leptin were a pill, it would be a diet pill. Normally, leptin acts directly on the hypothalamus, the part of the brain that controls the appetite. It both suppresses feelings of hunger and increases energy expenditure, the two ingredients needed for weight loss.

Adiponectin is another important hormone secreted by fat cells. This hormone is released after eating. Its main function is to regulate insulin sensitivity.[7] High blood levels protect against both heart attacks and diabetic complications associated with small blood vessel disease. Low levels, on the other hand, promote insulin resistance and blood vessel inflammation. Adiponectin is a plasma protein and, like all proteins, depends on a particular gene for its manufacture. Obese people, type 2 diabetics, and Zucker fatty rats all have low adiponectin levels because that particular gene, too, is mutated.

Zucker diabetic fatty rats (fa/fa) are obese because their double dose of mutant genes produces defective leptin; leptin that does not suppress hunger or attach it self to the walls of fat cells as it normally should. Thus, it cannot act as a selective key to allow fatty acids and triglycerides to freely enter *only* fat cells. Instead, the defective leptin permits fat to invade the tissues of organs where fat is not welcome. Fat cells don't belong in the liver, kidneys or pancreas. In these organs they interfere with normal function.

Some researchers contend that in humans, appetite suppression aside, leptin's primary function is to limit the storage of triglycerides (lipids, fats) to the normal anatomical fat stores, the fatty subcutaneous areas of the body, and to prevent storage of fat in other body regions where fat is usually absent.[8] Fat (or lipid) stored in fat cells (lipocytes) is readily available for use as fuel for energy. Misplaced fat, that stored in abnormal locations like the liver, muscle or pancreas functions only to disrupt normal physiology. If, for example, leptin fails to protect against fat accumulation in the beta cells of the pancreas, the result is beta cell malfunction. This translates into decreased insulin production and increased blood sugar levels — causing lipotoxic diabetes in rats.[9]

Research shows that obese people and those who have type 2 diabetes tend to accumulate fat cells in their pancreas, just like the experimental rats. The exact biochemical pathway for this pancreatic fat accumulation differs in humans, but the result is the same — beta-cell dysfunction and new onset or worsening diabetes. Inexplicably, the excess of leptin produced by the fatty tissue of type 2 diabetics (rats and humans) fails to enter the brain in sufficient quantities to suppress the appetite or to promote energetic activity, the two requirements for weight loss.[10] So obesity and type 2 diabetes have intertwined genetic origins. The genes for obesity produce ineffective leptin, the body's natural appetite suppressant. This results in weight gain in the form of fat accumulation, and fat cells (lipocytes) produces cytokines, the chemical substances that cause insulin resistance — the metabolic impairment responsible for type 2 diabetes. Therein resides a crucial (but not the only) pathological connection between obesity and type 2 diabetes.

But the quest for answers to our obesity problem gets even more complex. Our body fat is not the only non–glandular structure that acts like an endocrine gland. Recent research has identified our bony skeleton as yet another "endocrine gland." In this case, bone cells produce a hormone called osteocalcin. In the type 2 diabetic, osteocalcin and leptin have opposite functions. Osteocalcin normally acts as a regulator of glucose metabolism by increasing sensitivity and secretion of insulin. It promotes efficient sugar metabolism and, consequently, keeps the body lean. But this effect is negated by the diabetic's defective leptin, which fails to act as an appetite suppressant. The result, consequently, is weight gain.[11]

Genetic research is speeding up. Research methods have been streamlined by the modern biotechnology used to map the human genome, decode DNA, and clone research animals to serve as models for human disease (or obesity, as the case may be). But as progress is made in the field of obesity/type 2 diabetes research, new questions arise. The quest for answers becomes more complex. Genes are not as simple as they appear on paper. Their expression is intertwined with other genes, linked to multiple bodily functions, and often influenced by environmental factors such as our unlimited, twenty-first century industrialized food supply and our ever-decreasing need to expend energy.

In research jargon, genetically induced obesity is divided into three categories. The first type is monogenetic, where one gene is responsible. This is very rare. The second type is syndromic obesity, obesity linked to or associated with multiple specific anatomic and physiologic defects such as mental retardation, vision defects, sexual dysfunction, etc. This too is rare. The third and most common type is polygenetic obesity, defined as multiple genes on multiple chromosomes acting together to cause obesity, or acting separately, under the right environmental conditions, to make a person susceptible to obesity. Polygenetic factors are the cause of obesity in 40–70 percent of cases.[12] Indeed, genetic research has identified close to 600 "obesity genes," genes that affect weight loss or gain, or limit the expenditure of energy through disruption of normal metabolic pathways.[13]

Compounding the researchers' problems are the effect of the environment on specific genes (the epigenetic effect), difficulties in pooling various scientific conclusions in order to extract useful information, and making the jump from experimental animals to humans. You can grasp the complexity of reaching black-and-white answers regarding genetics and obesity. Nevertheless, you can be sure of two things: there is a genetic basis for obesity, and for 60 percent of Americans, that genetic underpinning is awakened by personal choices regarding eating habits and exercise. With all these genetic, physiologic and metabolic factors, you can argue that genes play a major role in obesity. Two people can share exactly the same diet, yet one may be thin and the other chubby. In America, genetics is a major factor in obesity and type 2 diabetes, but is it not true that many Americans have lost their sense of satiety — that they do not recognize when they have had enough to eat? In a little more than two hundred years our mindset has gone from Thomas Jefferson's sixth rule of living, "We seldom repent having eaten too little," to the McDonald's slogan, "Super-size me." Ultimately, the most effective method of conquering obesity is by controlling a single body part — the mouth! We eat too much, so we are a fat society; and fat societies are plagued with type 2 diabetes.

The Accidental Cure

The metabolic link between obesity and type 2 diabetes has been recognized for decades. As discussed above, it is assumed to be the result of an out-of-kilter metabolism caused by the gradual buildup of excess body fat. So the medical community and patients alike were taken by surprise when it became apparent that surgeons, of all people, could cure diabetes instantly with a simple weight-reduction operation. You would have thought such a feat would require pharmaceutical researchers or genetic engineers. After all, surgeons are not recognized as cognitive scientists. Had the cure been preceded by a well thought out theory and then proven in the operating room, we could take a bow. But alas, it was luck. Simple, unanticipated luck — like planting potatoes in your backyard and finding oil.

Weight-reduction surgery started out as just that — an operation designed to make patients thinner, more able to fit into (what was once) a sleek society. Surgeons knew from the start, thirty-five or forty years ago, that aside from the cosmetic effect, there were definite health benefits to weight-reduction surgery. The procedure relieved heart disease, sleep apnea, leg swelling, and chronic vein disease.

Early on, surgical complications were quite common. But as the operation grew in popularity, many kinks were eliminated, and newer, less invasive, laparoscopic techniques allowed for faster recovery. Because there is no shortage of morbidly obese patients to operate upon, some surgeons reduced their surgical repertoire. Now they could specialize, confine their practices to one procedure — weight-reduction surgery. The field of baro surgery was born.

At first, baro surgeons were thought of as opportunists. Obese people are common in our society. A surgical procedure can make them thin, and often their medical insurance doesn't cover it. The patient must pay out-of-pocket — and usually in advance. As an added bonus, weight reduction surgeons can live like gentlemen — nobody needs a 2 A.M. weight reduction operation. As demand for the procedure increased, so did the number of baro surgeons. Surgeons who were established in other, more work-intensive fields who had never before done the weight reduction procedure were offered two- or three-day training courses. Once "certified," they hopped on the bandwagon. Then, as the procedure became commonplace, a strange thing happened. Some previously unrecognized patient benefits came to light. Patients not only slimmed down and eliminated their sleep apnea and leg swelling, post-operative statistics indicated that their chances of developing many types of cancer had diminished, and, most surprising, their type 2 diabetes disappeared. It disappeared almost instantly, within days of the surgery.[14] No more pills, no more insulin, and the dreaded specter of diabetes-related heart disease, neuropathy, kidney failure, blindness and peripheral vascular disease had vanished.

Presently, metabolic surgery can be offered only to morbidly obese type 2 diabetics. It's considered unethical to perform weight loss surgery on a patient whose BMI is less than 40 or who is less than 100 lbs. overweight. The overweight but not morbidly obese type 2 diabetic or pre-diabetic can often achieve the same effect by losing 10 percent of his body weight — which is easier said than done. The key distinction between the surgery and dieting is the permanent weight loss attained by the surgery.

Suddenly, the baro surgeons had become vital members of the medical establishment. As word of the benefits of their operation spread, they puffed out their chests and took a new name — metabolic surgeons. They still don't have to work at night, and still usually get paid in advance.

But how could anyone have symptomatic, even insulin-dependent type 2 diabetes one day and be free of the disease the next? How, by simply rearranging the patient's anatomy, could the surgeon cure this disease? The answer can be found in the research lab, among the Zucker diabetic fatty rats.

The rapid response to surgery suggests that weight loss alone is not what cures the diabetes. These patients become non-diabetic even before the weight loss starts! There is an apparent "intestinal component" to type 2 diabetes, and the operation neutralizes it.[15] The exact diabetogenic intestinal component that is effectively eliminated by the surgery has not yet been defined, though there are several theories. If proven correct, these theories may lead to a simple surgery or even a pill to cure even the non-obese type 2 diabetic.

Bariatric surgery is effective. According to the combined results of several scientific studies involving 22,094 individuals, the average patient lost 62 percent of his body weight. Of those who underwent the simpler laparoscopic gastric banding procedure, 48 percent were cured of their type 2 diabetes. But patients who underwent the more extensive surgical gastric bypass procedure, where the duodenum is bypassed as well, were cured 84 percent of the time; and with an even more extensive operation, called a billiary-pancreatic diversion, 95 percent were cured of their type 2 diabetes. Lumped together, the various types of bariatric surgery cure 76.8 percent of patients of their type 2 diabetes. Additional benefits were a decrease in blood lipid levels (70 percent), curing or lessening high blood pressure (78.5 percent) and resolving or improving sleep apnea (87 percent).

Most surgeons (excluding metabolic surgeons) have a natural aversion to fat. That's not to say we don't care for heavy people; we simply don't enjoy operating on them. Operating on an obese patient is like gardening in the mud or driving in the fog. It makes the process slower and harder to navigate, and increases the probability of an undesirable outcome. Surgery is risky business. As a surgeon, one who attends weekly morbidity and mortality conferences, I can tell you that the true complication and mortality rates for bariatric surgery are significantly under-reported. The *alleged* re-operation rate for even the simplest of weight-reduction surgeries is estimated at only 6 percent, and when complications occur, they are serious.

Some advice: if bariatric surgery is recommended, seek an experienced metabolic surgeon, one who knows his (or her) field inside-out. With the introduction of complex surgical procedures and advanced surgical technologies, surgeons take longer to master their specialties. The American College of Surgeons, the credentialing organization for surgeons in the U.S., has encouraged surgeons to specialize. This is a good thing. If you are considering weight loss surgery and you meet the criteria, to decrease your chance of complications, have it done by an experienced bariatric surgeon, not a general or laparoscopic surgeon who performs the procedure only occasionally.[16]

Powerful genetic components control the metabolism of both Zucker rats and people, putting them all at risk for obesity. Those with an abundance of obesity-promoting genes must overcompensate — that is consume less food, expend more energy, and burn more calories in order to maintain a "normal" body weight. Legally, we say all men are created equal, but genetically they are not. In the final analysis it's both your eating habits and your genes that determine your size. The only controllable part of that equation is your eating habits.

In the United States, controlling your eating habits is difficult. The nutritional environment is appalling. Our children live amongst more than 200,000 fast food chain restaurants (aside from pizza parlors, hot dog stands and greasy spoons), where their often unsuspecting or nutritionally naive moms and dads ply them with inexpensive, fat-laden cheeseburgers, giant-sized sugary drinks, and fat-infused french fries. Parents shop in supermarkets and bodegas where the entrance to each aisle should be posted with a flashing neon sign: "Caution. Foods are Highly Processed — Added Sugar and Harmful Fats — Risk of Obesity and Diabetes! Enter at Your Own Risk!" Lifestyle for American children is not an option. It has been predetermined by one hundred years of industrialization.

Culture can have an enormous effect on body habitus. Women thought homely in one culture may be considered attractive in another. This is especially true in some Islamic countries of sub–Saharan Africa. In the small, northwest African country of Mauritania, for example, obese women are so revered that many Mauritanian mothers, in order to marry off their daughters, feel compelled to make them burqa-bursting fat. They force-feed their young girls gallon after gallon of camel's milk (there are no fast food restaurants in Mauritania). They even awaken them at night to meet their daily quota. Now, in order to fatten up their daughters for marriage, modern Mauritanian moms can take a scientific shortcut. On the display tables in the open-air Mauritanian markets, among the colorful cloths, salted snacks, dates, and desert fruits sit packets of Indian-made dexamethasone, a potent steroid, with no prescription needed. This drug, ordinarily used to treat serious inflammatory diseases, has a reliable though dangerous side effect. When taken regularly, it causes extreme obesity. Mauritanian men, of course, are the problem. They're not happy with thin or even slightly overweight women; for them, big really is beautiful.

Unfortunately, as we know, obesity leads to type 2 diabetes, cardiovascular disease, and various other weight-related health problems. According to a recent article in *The New York Times*, the women of Mauritania, influenced by western society, are starting to rebel.[17] The Mauritanian government, aware of the health dangers of obesity and the threat of type 2 diabetes, is encouraging mothers to allow their daughters to slim down.

Generation D, Childhood Type 2 Diabetes

Childhood obesity is a major risk factor for type 2 diabetes. My pediatrician colleagues will tell you they rarely saw type 2 diabetes twenty years ago, but today it's one of the most common new diagnoses in any pediatric practice. Here in America, urban children, it seems, no longer run around and play outside until dark. Their parents won't let them. Our changing world poses new risks to their safety. Parents must keep a watchful eye out. Children, obliged to be sedentary, sit and watch TV, surf the Web, or play video games. Many schools for want of funds have eliminated their physical education classes.

Childhood obesity and type 2 diabetes are not a uniquely American problem; they are a worldwide phenomenon. In Lisbon, Portugal, scientists studied nine- and ten-year-olds. They proved that the mere lack of vigorous physical activity (even in the absence of obesity) results in insulin resistance (the cause of type 2 diabetes).[18] If the kids are obese as well as sedentary, then the risk of developing type 2 diabetes is even greater. Eating habits and lack of exercise are only part of the problem. Type 2 diabetes in children, as determined through studies of the Arizona Pima Indians, is significantly increased if, as fetuses, the children were exposed to maternal diabetes.[19] There, in the womb, their metabolism is imprinted with the biochemical prerequisites to become diabetic. This association holds true for all racial groups and is independent of other risk factors like the mother's weight, father's history of diabetes, birth weight or even the child's obesity later in life. Furthermore, for all ethnicities, as social mores become more liberal and ethnic groups intermarry, our gene pool expands. Offspring of mixed ethnic couples are provided with additional genes, often the sleeping genes for type 2 diabetes. But it is our faulty eating habits and lack of exercise that awaken these genes and literally change the shape of American society.

Breastfeeding significantly reduces the odds of childhood obesity.[20] Pediatricians are taught early on to encourage new moms to breastfeed their babies. Aside from being the ideal nutrition for newborns, breast milk provides various immunological and general health benefits. Breastfeeding defines us. Mammals are higher vertebrates that nourish their young with breast milk. One benefit well proven but little known, is that breastfeeding significantly (13–22 percent) reduces the risks of both childhood and long term obesity. And breastfed babies are far less likely to develop type 2 diabetes later in life. This is true for the children of diabetic as well as non-diabetic mothers, and this benefit holds for the children of obese as well as non-obese mothers. The protective effect of breastfeeding is reduced when the mother supplements with formula and is enhanced proportionally as she continues to breastfeed exclusively. The American Academy of Pediatrics recommends breastfeeding through the first year of life.

Incidentally, there is one notable exception to the mammalian lock on breast feeding. There are three bird species that breastfeed: the mourning dove, the flamingo and the penguin. (The mourning dove gets its name from its plaintive call.) Doves, flamingos, and penguins have an interesting physical adaptation which is absent in other bird species. Through an opening in their breast feathers they provide their young with "pigeon's milk." These birds are anatomically unique. Like all birds they have a crop, a small pouch at the end of their esophagus, but unlike other birds, their crops communicate through a tube to an opening between the feathers in the skin of their breasts. The nourishing "pigeon's milk" is produced in the crops of both the male and female of these three bird species. The chicks suckle this "milk" directly through that breast opening. The crop milk, in fact, is somewhat similar to mammalian milk in that it's white and rich in protein and fat.

Type 2 diabetes in childhood and adolescence is difficult to detect and treat because symptoms may be minimal for the first few years. Children with type 1 diabetes, on the other hand, are prone to wide swings in their blood sugar levels. These drops in blood sugar may precipitate episodes of sweating, vomiting and confusion which may prompt panicky parental reactions and provoke trips to the emergency room. These experiences serve to remind the child with type 1 diabetes that self-management is extremely important, a concept that is difficult for type 2s to grasp.

Don't let the "2" in type 2 diabetes fool you; it doesn't mean less severe.[21] Research has shown that with the exception of retinopathy (eye problems), children and adolescents with type 2 diabetes have significantly more complications at an earlier age than children with type 1. Even though their disease may be present for a shorter time, type 2s are more likely to develop high blood pressure and the early onset of kidney disease, which is heralded by the appearance of protein in their urine. In addition, the high lipid and cholesterol levels in type 2 diabetic children and adolescents take their toll in later life as they progressively develop heart and peripheral vascular disease. Some investigators have found that the onset of neuropathy may occur earlier in the course of youth-onset type 2 diabetes than it does in children with type 1 diabetes.[22] These findings might well provide incentive for parents to help their adolescent children manage their disease if the parents are aware of the long-term consequences. Parents do know this — their kids don't appreciate the longterm consequences of their problem.[23] But then again, many newly diagnosed adults don't either.

Part Two

The Complications of Diabetes and How to Avoid Them

Chapter 4

GESTATIONAL DIABETES: THE CASE OF LUCKY LYDIA LANG

A lawsuit is a powerful memory stimulus. A doctor never forgets the circumstances surrounding a lawsuit, even if he is involved only as a witness. So the events of that Thursday when Lydia Lang showed up in the E.R. at one o'clock in the morning remain clear to me now, twenty years later. Back then, every senior surgeon took mandatory emergency room call. It was not unusual, when covering both general and vascular surgery, to see eight or ten acute surgical emergencies during a single 24-hour period. In our E.R., the beds are never empty. We have thirty acute-care beds; another eight or ten cots line the hallways, and a holding area temporarily houses the eighteen or twenty patients in need of observation, or awaiting admission.

Arriving patients are seen initially by the triage nurse, then by one of several shift-working E.R. physicians who evaluate them, then treats and releases his patient if the malady is minor. If the nature of the condition is not clear or the patient requires admission, he calls the appropriate specialist on duty that day. My 24-hour surgery call began Wednesday morning at 8 o'clock.

The day started out unusually quiet, with only an appendectomy early on, a couple of abscesses to be drained and the patients released, and of course, my already scheduled O.R. cases. I was home by 10 P.M., unwound with a snack and "The Late Show," and was in bed before midnight.

The phone woke me at 1:15 A.M. The E.R. clerk put me on hold for Dr. Lee. I waited, half asleep, until he picked up. There was no "Hello," or "Sorry to wake you." Night shift E.R. docs assume everyone is awake

73

and alert—after all, it's the middle of their day. I sat on the side of the bed, eyes closed, the phone to my ear. Then he began. "I've got a 43-year-old female diabetic with severe abdominal pain." He continued, "She weighs about 350 pounds. Her pain has been getting worse all day..." Wanting him to get to the point, I interrupted. "How long has she been in the E.R.?" There was silence while he read the chart.

Then he said, "She arrived at 10:30 P.M."

"What's she had done?" I asked.

"Well," he said. "She's had a chest X-ray, EKG, abdominal films, and the usual blood work."

"And?" I said, expecting to hear the results. "What did you find?"

"Well," he said, "the white cell count was 12,000 and the blood sugar was 300 mg. percent. We gave her ten units of insulin. Her other blood chemistries were okay; the urine had trace sugar and was positive for protein and ketones."

So, with that, I knew her diabetes was out of control; she was dehydrated, and probably had early kidney damage from her diabetes.

Then he added, "The abdominal films show multiple large, round calcifications. One of them's bigger than a softball. It looks like a fibroid uterus, but it's not a quality picture. She's huge!"

"Has she had a CAT scan?" I asked.

"No," he answered. "She refused; says she's claustrophobic. Anyway, I don't think she'd fit in the machine; she's too big."

"Where's her pain?" I asked, trying to make a telephone diagnosis, one that would save me a midnight run to the E.R. "Upper or lower abdomen, crampy or steady? Is there any blood in her urine?"

"The pain is all over," he said, "and yes, she has a trace of blood in her urine, but she says she's been spotting for months and doesn't have regular menstrual periods."

"Pregnancy test?" I asked.

"She says there's no way she could be pregnant. And she's got three kids with her, two teenage girls and a take-charge, twenty-something daughter."

"What was the gas pattern on her abdominal X-ray?" I asked, trying to rule out intestinal obstruction. I heard him thumb through the E.R. chart. He found the handwritten report on the X-ray slip and read: "Multiple large calcified pelvic masses consistent with fibroids, normal gas pattern in large bowel, suggest additional views."

"Did she have a pelvic ultrasound?" I asked.

"No," he responded. "I haven't called the ultrasound tech in yet. But I don't think she'll hold still for it; she's really uncomfortable. Should I call your resident?"

"No." I said. "Call GYN. It sounds like it's more in their territory than mine. Let me know — or ask the gynecologists to call me after they've evaluated her."

Sure, I was looking for an out, a reason to avoid a sleepless night saddled with someone else's problem. With a full O.R. day in front of me I would need to be alert. I'd convinced myself that she had a gynecological problem — the spotting, the crampy abdominal pain, yet a normal gas pattern and no fever. At least she would get a good pelvic exam; the E.R. doc didn't do one. I fell off to sleep.

There was no call back. My alarm went off at 5:50 A.M. I had half forgotten the call. Perhaps I was dreaming. I always dream that I'm working. Then, in the shower, the details of the conversation crystallized, and with them, a guilty notion. I should have gone in. Maybe I blew off a real surgical problem.

When I arrived at the hospital, I parked in the patients-only E.R. lot. I found Dr. Lee at the nurse's station; he was preparing to leave. "What happened to that lady?" I'd forgotten her name.

"Oh, Mrs. Lydia Lang," he said. "GYN took her — degenerating fibroids."

Fibroid tumors of the uterus are benign, but when they grow extremely large they begin to die in the center, like an over-ripe melon. As the dead area bleeds, the fibroid expands and this causes extreme pain. It's called "red degeneration."

"The GYN resident came down. He called Krinsky, he was the GYN attending on call. They took her to the O.R. They should be out by now."

"He never called me," I said.

"I know," said Lee. "He didn't want to wake you again, being it was a GYN problem."

Dr. Lee looked tired; his long night shift was finally over.

"Thanks," I said. "Get some sleep." My guilt vanished like a nurse when you need the bed-pan as I headed to the cafeteria for a cup of tea before my first case.

The only person in the doctor's eating area was Krinsky. He was sitting with his usual rosy-faced grin, still in his scrubs, his empty plate in front of him. I went over. "How're you doing?" I asked, knowing he'd been up all night.

"Ovary well," he quipped with a grin. "You?"

"Good," I said. "Thanks for not waking me again last night." With that, he pushed his chair back, snapped to mock attention, gave a half salute, and said, "At your cervix." Even at 7 A.M. he couldn't be serious. Then his pager went off. "Must be the recovery room," he said. "What do they want now? That case wasn't easy, you know — biggest fibroids I ever saw."

I did know; I saw the blood spatter on his scrub cap.

"What did you do?" I asked.

"A hysterectomy. What a uterus. We weighed it — fourteen and a half pounds."

He got up and pulled the receiver off the wall. "Krinsky," he announced. Then he listened for a few seconds and asked, "Who? Pathology ... OK, I'll call now ... OK right away, I'll call now." He dialed the extension, turned his back to me and spoke, but mostly listened. Then he came back to the table and flopped into his chair. The grin was gone. So was the rosy hue.

"Everything OK?" I asked. He looked down at his hands as if he had touched something dirty. "She was pregnant — she was in labor," he said. "That's what the pain was — contractions. The pathologist opened her uterus to see if the fibroids had bled and found a near-term fetus, a boy."

I thought to myself *how could they miss that, the X-ray?* Then it clicked — those calcified fibroids. Diabetics — they calcify everything. They must have mistaken the baby's head for one of the fibroids, and with her obesity obscuring the details, the other calcified fibroids hid the fetal bones. They'd have seen the fetus if she'd consented to the CAT scan or if they'd done an ultrasound.

I wondered if Dr. Lee had asked her about the possibility of being pregnant with the three kids in the room. She denied it. She might have known all along.

I felt bad for Krinsky. This was a lawsuit for sure. Thank God my name wasn't on the chart; in New Jersey that's enough to get you sued. I consoled Krinsky, told him he did what anyone would do. He nodded, his thoughts elsewhere.

Instead of going up to the O.R., I was already late, I went directly down to the pathology department. I had to see that uterus. Every surgical specimen is examined twice, when it first arrives, for the gross pathology, and then after the tissue is fixed, that is preserved in formaldehyde, when representative samples are taken for microscopic examination.

Dr. White, the pathologist handling the case, showed me the uterus. It was split open like one of those giant clam shells. The bluish-red placenta stuck, like the clam, to one half.

"Look at this thing," he said. "Have you ever seen fibroids like that? Beats me how she ever got pregnant. I've gotta be honest, when I opened it I gasped. I didn't expect this." He eyed the fetus.

The doll-sized, gray fetus, detached, but still curled up, was on a small, green O.R. towel in the center of a large, steel dissection table.

Pathology labs don't smell good, but this one was clothes-changing putrid. He saw me wince. "That's the amniotic fluid," he said. "Something's not right here."

I looked at the clock, ten to eight. "Gotta go, I'm late. Please call me with the results of the post; I'll be in the O.R."

It was near noon when I finished my first case. I was in the recovery room writing post-op orders with Frank, the intern, when Dr. White's number appeared on my pager. I punched his extension. He answered. "Good news," he said. "Or bad news — depends how you look at it. It appears this fetus died in utero, long before last night. He's got multiple congenital defects, including transposition of the great vessels and undeveloped lungs. This is a missed abortion."

I explained to Frank that a missed abortion is a pregnancy that ends with the death of the fetus, but the fetus remains in place.

"Did you call Krinsky?" I asked.

"Sure," he said, "but he's still upset about missing the diagnosis. He did the right operation for the wrong reason."

Of course she sued anyway. This is New Jersey, and as the two-story advertisement that's painted on the bricks of the building facing the hospital says: "If you've been mistreated by a physician, you may be entitled to..."

The case never went to trial. They settled out of court. I don't know for how much — or whether that was the worst day or the best day of Lydia Lang's life.

The Little Known, Long-Term Consequences of Gestational Diabetes

The case of Lydia Lang, assuming that she knew she was pregnant, demonstrates the worst-case scenario of unmonitored gestational diabetes.

Diabetes during pregnancy comes in two basic varieties: pre-existing diabetes (pre-gestational diabetes) and when a diabetic state develops during the pregnancy. In the United States, diabetes first recognized during a pregnancy (gestational diabetes) occurs 200,000 times each year. It affects about 8 percent of all pregnancies and up to 14 percent in high risk groups, according to the ADA. Routine testing for gestational diabetes is the norm in America. The diagnosis is made when a pregnant women's fasting blood sugar is over 140 mg/dl, or, if 2 hours after a 75 gram oral glucose challenge, the blood sugar level remains greater than 140 mg/dl.

In the past there was some question as to whether gestational diabetes was a disease or simply a normal physiologic reaction to pregnancy. Today, all experts in the care of diabetes consider it a serious disease, one that requires special treatment. This opinion is backed up by statistics showing that the incidence of maternal death (rare), high birth weight babies (macrosomia), shoulder dystocia (the baby's shoulder gets caught in the birth canal creating a surgical emergency), bone fractures, and nerve palsies resulting from difficult deliveries are considerably higher in the cases of mothers with gestational diabetes than in the cases of mothers with uncomplicated pregnancies. Moreover, if gestational diabetics are treated with dietary control, counseling and insulin when necessary, these complications can be reduced from 4 percent to 1 percent.[1]

Gestational diabetes is more likely to occur in overweight women over age thirty, and in women with a family history of diabetes. However, inexplicably, it occurs with some regularity in normal weight women who have no apparent risk factors. If diabetes is present before the pregnancy starts, the prospective mother is said to have pre-gestational diabetes. Prospective mothers with a history of type 2 diabetes (pre-gestational type 2 diabetics) tend to be older, more overweight, and to have been diabetic for a shorter time than women who have type 1 pre-gestational diabetes.

Every little bit of weight counts. The chance of developing gestational diabetes increases in direct proportion to the mother's weight. It is estimated that overweight women are twice as likely to develop gestational diabetes, obese women are four times as likely, and extremely obese women are eight times more likely to develop the condition.[2] Significantly, the risk of developing permanent type 2 diabetes also increases with the weight of the expectant mother.

Gestational diabetes is much more common in older moms, or perhaps older eggs. Today's medical technology allows young women's eggs to be removed, frozen and used years later for in-vitro fertilization. The risk of developing gestational diabetes increases progressively with the age of the pregnant mother. Studies have shown that mothers under twenty have a less than 2 percent chance of experiencing gestational diabetes. But a whopping 39 percent of mothers over forty develop gestational diabetes.[3] This impressive statistic has moved the American Diabetes Association to recommend that all pregnant women twenty-five or older be screened for gestational diabetes.

Women who've had gestational diabetes once tend to develop it again with future pregnancies. Most importantly, they have a 50/50 chance of developing permanent type 2 diabetes themselves within ten years.[4] The risk of developing permanent type 2 diabetes varies according to ethnicity. Asian women have the highest risk of developing gestational diabetes, closely followed by Hispanic women, then African Americans, then non–Hispanic Caucasian women.[5] The odds of developing permanent type 2 diabetes following gestational diabetes are even greater in women who require insulin treatment during their pregnancy. Half will develop type 2 diabetes within five years of giving birth. Across the board, according to the American Diabetes Association, the overall, longterm, risk of these women developing permanent type 2 diabetes exceeds 70 percent. Unfortunately, most women with gestational diabetes do not grasp this fact.[6] They do realize that gestational diabetes may well be a harbinger of permanent diabetes, but they don't consider themselves among the high-risk group.

Compounding this problem is the failure of many primary physicians and gynecologists to follow up. Records show that many of these doctors do not regularly screen for pre-diabetes or for the onset of type 2 diabetes. In addition, few of them counsel their gestational diabetic patients in the weeks, months, and years following delivery.

Occasionally, type 1 diabetes can occur following a gestational pregnancy, but this is apparently not related to the metabolic derangements of the pregnancy. Ninety-nine percent of women who develop diabetes following a gestational diabetic pregnancy get type 2.

During pregnancy, the mother's pancreas produces more insulin. However, her placental hormones counteract the glucose-lowering effect of the increased insulin. The placenta, like the body's fat and bone, behaves like another one of those "giant endocrine glands." It secretes hormones and cytokines, both of which cause insulin resistance, making blood sugars climb. In turn, the mother's insulin requirements and output are increased. By the end of an uncomplicated, normal pregnancy, blood

insulin levels are double those of a non-pregnant woman. Gestational diabetes appears when the blood sugar stays high because the mother's pancreas tires out, and the need for more and more insulin cannot be met.

Fetal growth requires insulin, too. Sugar-laden maternal blood flows
through the placenta and into the fetus. In order to utilize this excess
sugar, the fetus steps up insulin output. The nutritive effect of the mother's
high blood sugar on the developing fetus causes too rapid fetal growth,
and that results in big babies, macrosomia. Large babies translate into
difficult deliveries, so with gestational diabetes both the caesarian section
rate and the need for early pharmacologic induction of labor is increased.
In short, gestational diabetic women have large babies because the nutritive effect of the mother's too-high blood sugar coursing through the placenta continually overfeeds the developing fetus.

Pre-eclampsia is a common pathologic condition in pregnancy. It is
characterized by high blood pressure and the appearance of protein in the
expectant mother's urine. It occurs more frequently in gestational and pre-
gestational diabetics than in non-diabetic women. Lydia Lang had this
condition, though it was not recognized. She had hypertension and protein in her urine. Pre-eclampsia may occur in normal pregnancies, too,
and has been recognized, even in the absence of gestational diabetes, as
yet another significant risk factor for the mother's future development of
type 2 diabetes.

For good reason, birth defects are rare in gestational diabetes. This
is because anatomic fetal development is already complete by the end of
the third month and gestational diabetes usually does not appear until
after the fourth month. On the other hand, pregnant pre-gestational type
2 diabetics and pregnant type 1 diabetics have high blood sugars from the
start. So during the first three months of the pregnancy, while fetal development is in progress, abnormally high blood sugar levels may cause birth
defects. And with pre-gestational diabetes, high blood sugars throughout
the pregnancy compound the chance of large babies (11, 12, 13 pounds),
still births, and cesarean sections. In order to avoid these problems, pre-
gestational and gestational diabetics require close monitoring and tight
control of their blood sugar throughout their pregnancy. Diabetes in pregnancy is a serious condition; consultation with a diabetes specialist or an
obstetrician who deals with high-risk pregnancies reduces the chance of
complications from gestational diabetes.

Immediately following delivery, for the mother, all signs of gestational diabetes disappear (as we know, this may be temporary). The baby,

as a result of its high insulin levels while still in the womb, may be born with a dangerously low blood sugar. So, the newborn may need temporary treatment with intravenous glucose. The children of gestational diabetic women have a pronounced predisposition to become obese and diabetic. Thus, a vicious cycle is set in motion, one that insures the occurrence of type 2 diabetes in generation after generation. Several theories attempt to explain why the offspring of diabetic mothers are so prone to develop diabetes. One theory suggests it's a purely genetic phenomenon. Another implicates the altered intrauterine milieu in which the fetus develops — one in which the mother's high glucose levels and altered placental hormone levels give rise to permanent changes in the offspring's insulin metabolism. As the gestational diabetic's fetus develops in a high glucose environment, it becomes imprinted with the metabolic pathways that lead to type 2 diabetes.[7] Oversimplified: if you put a cucumber in the pickle barrel, you get another pickle. But chances are the transmission of diabetes across generations has multiple causes: genes, maternal imprinting, and the effect of our artificial environment. For now, researchers agree, the only way to break the cycle is to control the pregnant mother's weight and carefully monitor her glucose levels.

Here in the United States, the incidence of gestational diabetes is increasing dramatically, a direct result of the growing problems of obesity, older maternal age, and sedentary lifestyles. Increasing immigration of high-risk ethnic groups and their adoption of the American lifestyle puts immigrants near the top of the list for gestational diabetes. But for all groups, it is generally accepted that obesity, a high body mass index (BMI), is *the* major risk factor.

The likelihood of redeveloping gestational diabetes with second or third pregnancies can be reduced if prior to becoming pregnant again the mother can reduce her weight and achieve a normal body mass index. Studies confirm that one way to achieve this weight loss is by reducing consumption of foods which greatly elevate the blood sugar levels. We read the box to see what we're eating. Accurate listing of nutritional facts on packaged foods is important, but it's often confusing and sometimes outright misleading. For example, the nutritional value charts on two different types of breakfast cereal may be identical, but the actual effect on your blood sugar may be quite different.

Some foods, like white rice, will give you a quick spike in blood sugar levels, but others, like brown rice, may have the same calorie count but they elevate your blood sugar slowly and, in some cases, keep it up longer.

Foods that raise your blood sugar rapidly are said to have a high *glycemic index*. Those that raise your blood sugar slowly are said to have a low glycemic index. These effects may be important, especially for insulin-dependent diabetics or type one diabetics whose blood sugars tend to rise or fall rapidly. Gestational diabetes may benefit from recent research that indicates "a low-glycemic index diet significantly reduces the need for insulin" in gestational diabetes.[8] But the nutritional/metabolic implications are not as simple as white bread with its high glycemic index or lettuce with its low glycemic index. Processed foods are complex and their glycemic indices are difficult to gauge. Aside from that, food manufacturers are not shy about trying to fool you. They manipulate the numbers. Cheerios, for instance, sells its product plain or sugar-coated, but the calorie count is listed as 100 calories per serving for both types. In small print the manufacturer discloses that the serving size is smaller, 3/4 cup rather than 1 cup, for the sugar-coated variety. The metabolic implications, the glycemic index, is not a part of the nutritional chart.

Processed foods, those with additives, alterations, and multiple ingredients are higher in calories and glycemic index than natural foods. Unfortunately, supermarket shelves are filled with processed foods. The cereal manufacturers know that portion size is the fundamental factor in weight gain; that's why they don't emphasize it on the box. Reduced portion size is what weight control programs rely upon to be effective. Reduced portion size is also the reason that stomach stapling and other weight reduction surgeries are so effective. These surgical procedures drastically reduce the stomach size (and, in effect, the portion size). After a few bites the patient feels full. There's no way to overeat.

Dietary fiber, it is alleged, reduces the incidence of gestational diabetes.[9] Dietary fiber is that part of any planted or harvested food product — fruits, vegetables, and nuts — that holds the cells composing that food together and gives it structure. Fiber is not digestible by humans. Pandas can digest fiber. They eat only bamboo. They have specialized digestive enzymes and micro organisms that we lack. But fiber is good for us and may be particularly good for pregnant women. According to one study, eating about fifty grams, a little less than an ounce of fiber a day, significantly lowers glucose levels in the blood, thus improving insulin levels. Increasing fiber intake has been suggested, but not proven to decrease the likelihood of developing gestational diabetes. The American Diabetes Association in fact suggests that high fiber diets hold no benefit in glucose control.[10] Gestational diabetes, in many cases, is nutritional in origin, but avoiding it is not all that simple. If you've had or have gestational diabetes, I would advise that you see a certified nutritionist. Every hospital has a few.

Exercise is good for pregnant women.[11] Regular exercise lowers blood sugar and helps control weight by burning off calories. Research has shown that regular exercise is not only beneficial in diabetic control, it also reduces the risk of developing gestational diabetes. Studies and physician surveys show that obstetricians are soft in advising their patients to exercise. If there are no medical reasons to avoid exercise during pregnancy, it should be a regular routine. It's a proven method of keeping blood sugar down.

Women with gestational diabetes need to know that they are at significant risk to develop permanent diabetes and, eventually, its complications. They cannot afford to take a wait-and-see attitude. The American Diabetes Association recommends that "women with gestational diabetes should be screened for diabetes six weeks postpartum (after delivery) and should be followed up with subsequent screening for the development of diabetes or pre-diabetes." But physicians can be lax; recommendations for prevention — and following them — are two different stories. There is no magic bullet, no pill, and no genetic intervention. Experts in the field of gestational diabetes agree that the afflicted mother "needs to become aware of the benefits of modest weight loss and participating in regular physical activity, and [that] monitoring for the appearance of [pre-diabetes or type 2] diabetes should be preformed every one to two years."[12]

In the final analysis, it is clear that the rising incidence of gestational diabetes is not only a major cause of permanent diabetes in the afflicted mother, it triggers a chain reaction as well — a chain reaction that can lead to type 2 diabetes her children and her children's children, generation after generation.

Chapter 5

NEUROPATHY, THE
MOST COMMON
DIABETIC COMPLICATION

We are not solar powered. We require oxygen and nutrients to keep us alive, but like the Energizer Bunny, we are powered by electricity. Every step we take, every move we make, every heartbeat, every breath, every bodily function from digestion to dreaming is powered by electricity. When we think *electricity*, we think of Thomas Edison and the electric light. We picture electricity generated by electrons moving along a wire from one point to another as a current. The electricity that runs our bodies comes in the form of electronically charged metallic molecules of potassium (K), sodium (Na), chloride (CL), and calcium (Ca) that reside in our body fluids. The electricity in our bodies is biochemical electricity, akin to the chemical electricity produced by a car battery or a flashlight.

The most obvious example of biologically generated electricity is the current produced by the electric eel. It immobilizes its prey by electrocuting it. The electric eel can generate up to 1,000 volts, enough to light a lamp, stun a horse, or kill a large fish with one bite.

Our biologic, ion-generated electricity is just as real as Edison's electron-generated electricity. Both types have similar features and both are measured in volts. While Edison's electricity is composed of electrons traveling along metal wires, our biologic electricity is conducted by electrolytes, positively and negatively charged metals that are dissolved in our body fluids. In our bodies, the wires are long nerves, bundles of fibers, some pencil size, some microscopic, all composed of specialized nerve cells. The nerve fibers are connected in tandem by junctions called synapses. Our nerves are covered by insulating sheaths made of a white lipoprotein material called myelin. The myelin sheaths function like the plastic covering of the electric cords of appliances that you plug into your wall sockets. These sheaths prevent the electric current from disbursing and keep it flowing in one direction.

Our nervous systems are quite vulnerable to the deranged metabolism of diabetes. Nerve cell damage, the most common diabetic complication, is called *neuropathy*. The severity of neuropathy is clearly related to the length of time you have diabetes and how well the disease is controlled. Persistent high blood sugar levels damage nerve cells, and the myelin sheaths can be damaged by a lack of oxygen supply or by defects in the diabetic's lipoprotein metabolism.[1]

Our nervous systems are more complex than any computer. Simply defined, we have a central monitoring system — the brain and spinal cord — and three types of peripheral nerves: sensory nerves, motor nerves and autonomic nerves. All three can be affected by neuropathy.

Our sensory nerves allow us to appreciate external and internal sensations: pain, touch, taste, smell, position sense (proprioception), and hearing. The basic mechanism for the sensory system is a myriad of relays. Consider the complex circuitry of a painful finger prick. First there is an electric transmission from the injured skin to the spinal cord and then back to the injured area — that circuit takes a nanosecond and sets off a reflex motor nerve reaction to pull the finger from the painful prick. Then we experience a conscious emotional reaction, a chemical/neuronal reaction, in the brain, telling us what to do next. This complex bio-electric circuitry is basic to all vertebrates, and, as it happens, is an easy target at every level for the deranged metabolism of the diabetic.

Our motor nervous system facilitates voluntary physical actions: making a fist, chewing, walking, etc. Motor nerves, like sensory nerves, require input from the central nervous system, the brain and spinal cord, in order to function properly.

The autonomic (automatic) nervous system mediates physiologic activities: sweating, thinking, digestion, thought processes and emotions. It runs on electricity, too. But in order to function properly, the autonomic nervous system combines electrical activity with the release of chemical transmitters: acetylcholine, epinephrine, serotonin, histamine and others. In this neurological system, the electric circuitry is transformed; some of the synapses are modified to release these chemical messengers rather than to function as simple electrical transfer switches. The autonomic nervous system is responsible for the activity of endocrine glands; it can affect your heart rate or your blood pressure, produce tears, give you hives, make you blush, make you sweat, or give you nightmares. It is the part of our nervous system that distinguishes us from robots.

Nerves, like all living tissues, require oxygen for survival. In the diabetic patient, delivery of oxygen to vital tissues can be disrupted in two ways. One way is by atherosclerotic obstruction of the pipeline, the major oxygen-carrying arteries to the legs, kidneys or brain. Another way is by damage to oxygen-delivering capillaries. The capillaries normally function as selectively permeable membranes. They release oxygen from hemoglobin molecules like tea from tea bags, and take in metabolic waste products, including carbon dioxide, like a plant's roots absorb water. In the diabetic, damage to the capillaries is called *microangiopathy*, or small vessel disease.

A quick review of the circulatory system will clarify this. The heart receives oxygenated blood from the lungs. The oxygenated blood is pumped out of the left ventricle via the arteries, which gradually decrease in size, ultimately becoming barely visible arterioles. The arterioles shrink further to become thin-walled capillaries. The thin-walled capillaries transfer the oxygen carried by hemoglobin molecules in red blood cells to the body's tissues. At the same time, carbon dioxide (waste) is drawn into the capillaries. The capillaries then enlarge and become veinules. The veinules further enlarge to become veins that carry oxygen-poor, carbon dioxide-rich blood back to the heart's right ventricle, which then pumps it to the lungs where the carbon dioxide is exhaled and oxygen is taken in — then the cycle starts again. The lungs are also powered by electricity, which is transmitted simultaneously along the two phrenic nerves. These nerves supply power to the diaphragm, which is really two muscles, one on the left and one on the right, that act like a bellows. The phrenic nerves run from the cervical spine, down the neck, through the chest, and over the heart to the surface of the diaphragm. For some reason the phrenic nerves are not affected by diabetic neuropathy. But polio, Lou Gehrig's disease, venomous snake bites, brainstem strokes, and careless surgeons can damage one or both phrenic nerves and make breathing impossible.

In the diabetic, the fundamental exchange of blood gases through the capillary wall — oxygen to the tissues, carbon dioxide back to the lungs — may be disrupted. As diabetes progresses, microangiopathy becomes more prominent. Subtle changes take place in the cellular architecture of the capillary walls; they become thicker and less permeable, allowing too little oxygen to reach the myelinated nerves. Neuropathy ensues. At the same time, the already delicate capillary wall weakens further. This results in a tendency for the hair-like vessels to rupture and bleed. When capillaries rupture in the eye's retina, the bleeding is readily observed through an ophthalmoscope. Diabetic microangiopathy is a major cause of neuropathy and is, in part, responsible for visual impairment from retinal hemorrhaging, poor wound healing, diminished brain function, and kidney failure as well.

All three types of nerves — sensory, motor, and autonomic — may be affected by diabetic neuropathy. The first nerves affected are usually the peripheral sensory nerves of the feet and lower legs. It starts as numbness, or a pins-and-needles sensation. As time passes, the condition progresses to total loss of pain sensation in the feet. Some diabetics, up to 33 percent in some scientific studies, experience sensory neuropathy as severe, chronic, burning foot pain, a condition for which there is little effective relief.[2] Sensory neuropathy is a major cause of diabetic foot ulceration, especially when combined with motor neuropathy involving the muscles contained within the foot, the intrinsic foot muscles. Without a motor nerve supply, the muscles atrophy and the toes become cocked-up. The foot becomes claw-like. As a result, the patient walks with the pressure redistributed to the balls of his feet, and, lacking pain sensation, cannot feel the trauma. This leads to ulceration over the bony prominences, the metatarsal heads. In addition to sensory and motor neuropathy, autonomic neuropathy can target the sweat glands, causing dry, cracked skin, especially in the heels. To prevent this source of ulceration, it is imperative to keep the skin of the feet supple with emollients. This is discussed below.

One of my type 2 diabetic patients, a practicing physician with profound sensory and motor neuropathy, developed an ulceration on the ball of his right foot. Infection soon followed. His lack of pain delayed the urge to seek prompt medical attention. The infection progressed to involve the bones; he developed osteomyelitis. In spite of his longstanding diabetes and advanced neuropathy, his leg circulation was quite good. Though neuropathy and circulatory impairment often appear together, they are separate processes. By the time I saw him, his foot was so badly infected that despite receiving potent intravenous antibiotics and extensive surgical debredement (removal of dead tissue), he required a right-sided, below-the-knee amputation. This was his only option.

In view of his severe peripheral neuropathy, in an effort to preserve his remaining foot, his diabetologist and I took him to a well-known maker of form-fitted shoes. His plan was to make an exact plaster mold of my patient's neuropathic left foot and then, with the mold in hand, make a precisely fitting, soft leather shoe with no pressure points. This would safeguard the remaining foot. When we arrived, his diabetologist and I observed the plaster mold procedure. Our diabetic physician friend was given a seat and told to remove his shoe and sock. As he slipped the shoe from his foot, out tumbled thirty-five cents in small change; he'd been walking on the coins all day. He never felt a thing.

In decades past, advanced syphilis was the major cause of neuropathy. Today it's type 2 diabetes. Neuropathy may appear in non-diabetics as a complication of B-vitamin deficiency. It can complicate Celiac disease, a genetically acquired, autoimmune disease that affects 10 percent of the U.S. population. Celiac disease is an intestinal disorder set in motion by the ingestion of gluten, a component in all wheat products. This is why there are so many wheat-free products on supermarket shelves. Neuropathy is often a side effect of chemotherapy, particularly of those agents related to Taxol, often used in breast cancer therapy. *Idiopathic neuropathy,* a condition we see from time to time, means the loss of pain sensation without apparent cause. (*Idiopathic* is a medical term for "we have no clue.")

Occasionally I encounter yet-to-be-diagnosed pre-diabetics who complain of tingling in the feet or loss of pain sensation in the toes. When tested, they indeed have impaired glucose tolerance (glucose tolerance tests that fall in the range of 120 to 126 mg percent). Skin biopsies done on these patients may reveal a decreased density of intra-epidermal nerve fibers, a microscopic finding that verifies the presence of neuropathy in the pre-diabetic.[3] This is important, because when these pre-diabetic patients are placed on a proper diet and receive exercise counseling and proper medications to lower their blood pressure, blood sugar, and cholesterol, their neuropathy may lessen or disappear, and the onset of diabetes may be delayed or eliminated.

Medications are available for treatment of sensory neuropathy. Neurontin (gabapentin), a drug that was designed to treat epilepsy, is often prescribed, but patient feedback is not encouraging. The drug's effectiveness is questionable and its side effect, drowsiness, may interfere with daily activities. The best way for diabetics to minimize the symptoms of neuropathy is to keep their blood sugars normal and wear supportive, soft leather shoes.

Motor neuropathy, the second type of diabetic nerve damage, manifests itself as a specific loss of muscle function, a bioelectric power failure. Aside from affecting the muscles within the foot, motor neuropathy commonly affects the peroneal nerve, the power source for the extensor muscles of the foot. The result is a "foot-drop"—an inability, at the ankle joint, to extend the foot upward. The toes drag on the ground with each step. The patient compensates by lifting the affected foot higher with each step. This condition is not unique to diabetics; it can also result from alcoholism or trauma. The remedy for foot-drop is to provide the patient with a plastic foot brace. This keeps the ankle joint at a proper angle, so the foot won't drag when walking.

"Wrist-drop" is another example of motor neuropathy. Here, the radial nerve, one of three major nerves in the arm, becomes nonfunctional. The result is an inability to cock up the wrist as when gesturing "stop!" The treatment, a wrist splint, enables near-normal function. Bells palsy, paralysis of the facial muscles on one side, is a debilitating peripheral motor neuropathy of the facial nerve. It occurs in diabetics, but more often it's the result of other conditions: Lyme disease, idiopathic (unknown cause), or intentional (or unintentional) sacrifice during surgery of the parotid salivary gland through which the facial nerve passes.

An interesting neuropathic deformity is Charcot foot. Jean Charcot was a nineteenth-century French neurologist. He first described this deformity in patients with advanced syphilis, but today the most common cause is diabetic neuropathy. Here, the foot becomes misshapen from slippage, micro-fractures, and misalignment of the bones. When the process begins, multiple micro fractures cause the foot to swell and become inflamed. In this acute phase, Charcot foot can be misdiagnosed as an acute foot infection. This may lead to inappropriate treatment with antibiotics, attempted drainage—even amputation. Simple X-ray examination may only confuse the issue. Careful physical examination is the key to making the correct diagnosis. If no opening in the skin can be found, no port of entry for bacteria, then in spite of the infected appearance, infection is not likely. The proper treatment for Charcot foot is rest, taking the weight off the foot during the acute phase. As time passes, the swelling and redness subside, but deformity remains. Both of these deformities, cocked-up toes and Charcot foot, require form-fitted shoes in order to avoid ulceration.

In Diabetes, Elective Foot Surgery Is a Mistake

There is no justification for prophylactic or cosmetic foot surgery in the diabetic. Any foot deformity, especially one accompanied by motor/

sensory nerve impairment, is vulnerable to ulceration. It is vital for diabetics to understand that bunions and hammer toes, although unsightly, should not be operated upon unless they've progressed to ulceration. For all diabetics, newly diagnosed or longstanding, the risk of developing a non-healing surgical wound or infection far outweighs the benefit of elective foot surgery. Misshapen feet should be accommodated with form-fitted shoes. Unfortunately, many diabetics end up in the vascular surgeon's office after an ill advised elective podiatric procedure.

Autonomic neuropathy, the third type of diabetic nerve damage, is most interesting and quite debilitating. One example, gastric atony (gastroparesis), involves loss of electric power to the nerves controlling the muscular stomach wall. As a result, the stomach becomes flaccid. Food can not be propelled into the small intestine; the stomach remains full. The patient develops nausea, abdominal bloating, acid reflux, vomiting, and the feeling of having eaten too much even after having eaten little. Ordinarily, the muscular stomach walls push food on into the small intestine in a matter of minutes or hours; with gastric atony, food sits in the stomach for days. This can be a vexing problem. Fortunately, the condition usually responds to a day or two of fasting supplemented by intravenous fluids. But occasionally (in less than one in five cases) the condition requires surgical placement of a feeding tube into the small intestine below the bloated stomach.

Gastroparesis is more common in type 1 diabetics than in type 2s. It is not a condition unique to diabetics; almost half the cases appear in non-diabetics. People with gastroparesis are prone to depression and the development of gallstones.[4] Occasionally the accumulated vegetable matter congeals and forms a ball of undigested food, a bezoar. Bezoars can grow to the size of basketballs. When they can't escape the stomach they require open surgical removal.

Autonomic neuropathy involving the cardiovascular system is common and serious. It affects primarily the type 1 diabetic, but type 2s, after years with the disease, may eventually develop cardiac neuropathy, too. The electrical conduction system of the heart determines the number of beats per minute and the rhythm of the heart beat. Advanced cardiac autonomic neuropathy may inhibit the ability to generate a rapid heart beat when the heart is physically stressed, thereby curtailing the ability to exercise. In addition, loss of pain sensation results in silent heart attacks. They show up on EKG without ever having caused symptoms. Changes in cardiac rhythm (cardiac arrhythmias), may result in sudden death from the ineffective pumping of blood to vital organs. Cardiac autonomic neuropathy may be readily detected by your physician if, during an EKG examination, he observes the lack of heart rate variation in response to deep breathing. But it may go by unnoticed; doctors are so over-dependent on technology these days that a thorough physical examination is a rarity.

Patients with longstanding diabetes may lose the urge to urinate. A neurogenic bladder, one that will not empty on command, is not uncommon. I see patients who can pass urine only by pressing down on their lower abdomen with both hands; they manually squeeze the urine out. Most people with a severe neurogenic bladder have no choice but to self-catheterize several times a day. If they leave the catheter in the bladder continuously (an indwelling urinary catheter), they put themselves at substantial risk of developing a urinary tract infection.

Neurogenic bladder, the inability to release urine, most often affects men. Female diabetics, on the other hand, have quite the opposite problem; they can't hold it in. They're prone to urinary incontinence. Interestingly, obese Caucasian diabetic women have the highest incidence; more than one in four are affected. Non-Caucasian Hispanic, African American and Asian women, for some reason, are rarely troubled by this complication. They have about the same risk of incontinence as their non-diabetic counterparts.[5]

But the most common form of diabetic autonomic nerve damage is loss of sweat gland function in the feet. The result is dry skin which cracks and fissures easily. The heels are most affected. Loss of sweat gland function can occur with normal or impaired pain sensation and with normal or impaired circulation. When skin fissures complicate poor circulation they are extremely painful and often progress to infection, which can lead to — well, you know the story.

All diabetics, whether they have loss of sweat gland function or not, would be wise to keep their feet supple by using a skin emollient. The daily application of cocoa butter or lanoline used sparingly and not between the toes is most effective. Diabetics should never soak their feet. Foot soaking may feel good, but it results in tissue damage, much in the same way frequent contact with dishwater results in dishpan hands. Physicians who know diabetes well will never suggest foot soaking or, for that matter, prescribe whirlpool treatments.

Diabetics are extremely prone to oral cavity disease. They're troubled with gum disease and periodontal abscesses. Frequently, neuropathy of the oral cavity causes dry mouth (xerostomia), a burning sensation in the tongue (glosssodynia), and even trouble swallowing (see Chapter 11).

Pathologic alteration of the human electrical system, neuropathy, is the most common complication of diabetes. All living matter, in fact, depends on electricity for survival. Over 100 years ago, the pioneering Indian biophysicist Jagadis Chandra Bose (1858–1937) proved that even plants run on electricity.[6] Plants have no nerves or filaments to carry the electric charge; instead, their cell membranes pass electrically charged ions of calcium, chlorine and potassium from one cell to the next. This results in a tiny but measurable electric current which produces alterations in cell turgor (swelling). Electrically stimulated transient swelling (+) and contraction (–) of plant cells is responsible for basic plant physiology. Bose chose the most obvious examples for his experiments. He used certain species of Mimosa, whose sensitive leaves and stems dip and droop when touched or otherwise stimulated, a turnoff for animals who want to eat them; and Desmodium, a Himalayan plant whose leaves have a natural tendency to gyrate rhythmically.

Just as our nervous systems are set into motion by our five senses responding to internal and external stimuli, so it is with plants whose electrical activity (nervous system) is inextricably bound to environmental stimuli — sunlight, temperature, etc. Bose proved that the ascent of tree sap in the spring (the time for collecting maple syrup) and its descent in the fall are bioelectrical phenomena. He determined that a minute electric current produces an alternation of plant cell turgor and relaxation; this results in a hydraulic wave that propels the sap upward each spring.

Bose's extensive experimentation in plant physiology revealed some remarkable parallels to the human nervous system. In one instance, he amputated the leafy stems of Himalayan Desmodium plants, intentionally interrupting the electric current to the flapping leaves. They fell limp. Then he applied a weak electrical stimulus to the severed ends and the leaves once again began to flap. Had he cut a human nerve, say the radial, which controls motion at the wrist, he would have produced the same deficit. The wrist would have become limp, but an electrical stimulus applied to the cut nerve end would reestablish function. The same electronic principle is employed in the mechanism of cardiac pacemakers, modern bioelectric limb prostheses, and defibrillators.

Since Bose's time, twenty-first century science has refined the instrumentation for measuring electrical potential and has developed the electron microscope. Yet modern science has not refuted his original findings; it has only confirmed and refined them.

Incidentally, it was Bose's experimentation with electromagnetic radiation that resulted in the invention of a device for recovering microwaves. This device, slightly altered, was used by Marconi without crediting Bose to receive the first transatlantic wireless radio signals in 1901.

Chapter 6

PERIPHERAL VASCULAR DISEASE: THE CASE OF ANNIE WALKER

Rabbits, the ultimate vegetarians, do not get clogged arteries.[1] Arthrosclerosis is simply not part of their ageing process. That's why, in 1908, the Russian researcher A.I. Ignatowski chose rabbits to prove his groundbreaking theory: that something in the human diet was responsible for the gradual clogging of our arteries. Dr. Ignatowski's experiments define the very basis of cardiovascular disease, yet ask any physician who he is and, chances are, the physician will never have heard of him. Dr. Ignatowski fed his experimental rabbits meat and eggs, and — that's right — the pink, silky-smooth lining of their arteries turned to yellow cobblestone. They all developed rampant atherosclerosis.

Shortly after this discovery, Nicholi Anichkov, a Russian doctoral student, with Ignatowski's rabbits in mind began writing his doctoral thesis. In 1912, Anichkov presented proof that certain cells within arterial walls gobble up a particular substance — cholesterol. After receiving his doctorate, Anichkov and his team fed pure cholesterol to their rabbits; their findings led them to accurately describe the cellular and physiologic basis of atherosclerosis. In 1950, Dr. John Gofman's experiments confirmed these findings. It was Dr. Gofman who, in 1951, using high speed centrifuges, spun down the cholesterol-laden blood serum from his carnivorous rabbits. He found two components: high density (HDL) and low density (LDL) cholesterol.

Dr. Gofman's group went on to prove that low density cholesterol (LDL) is responsible for the acceleration of atherosclerosis in human beings. In 1952, Dr. Laurence Kinsell proved that eating fruits and vegetables while avoiding animal fats significantly lowered blood cholesterol levels. Further research confirmed that a diet high in vegetable fats (unsaturated fats) has a cholesterol-lowering effect. With one exception, ever since these discoveries, the food industry has included cholesterol and unsaturated fat content information on its packaging labels. Ironically, that exception is egg cartons, and, incidentally, there are 200 mg. of cholesterol per egg yolk.

Two separate processes take place in ageing arteries — both are accelerated in the type 2 diabetic. The first is *arteriosclerosis*, or calcification of the artery wall, and the second, described above, is *atherosclerosis*, the buildup of plaque within the arterial lumen. The Greek derivation of the word atherosclerosis is *athera*, meaning gruel or porridge, and *skleros*, meaning hard. Arteriosclerosis and atherosclerosis are part of our normal ageing process. A major characteristic of type 2 diabetes mellitus is high levels of low density cholesterol (hypercholesterolemia).

In other words, in the arteries of the diabetics there are two processes going on simultaneously: hardening of the artery wall with calcium, and plugging of the lumen, the channel, with atharoma or plaque. Plaque is made up of lipoproteins, triglycerides, and cholesterol. Cholesterol is the major component. The two types, as we know from Dr. Gofman's research, are LDL, low-density lipoprotein (lousy, or bad cholesterol), and HDL, high density lipoprotein (happy, or good cholesterol). LDL cholesterol is bad because it acts like saturated fat; it builds up on the inner surface of your blood vessel walls. HDL cholesterol is good because it attaches itself to the bad cholesterol in your bloodstream, and prevents it from accumulating on the inner walls of your arteries. Then it filters out through the liver, where it is broken down and excreted in the bile. Thickening of the blood vessel walls, arterial occlusive disease, is the process responsible for most diabetic complications: kidney disease, loss of vision, heart attack, stroke, and diabetic foot problems, which often lead to amputation. And neuropathy, the most common diabetic complication is, in part, due to thickening of blood vessels, which cuts the oxygen supply to sensory nerves and their sheaths.

Cholesterol makes the evening news, while triglycerides, just as important, keep a low profile. A high triglyceride (fat) level in the blood (above 200 mg/dl) is typical of type 2 diabetes. In the human body triglycerides take two forms: liquid in the blood or solid, as body fat. Body fat is 99 percent triglyceride and serves two basic needs: it's a major source of energy and it insulates, preventing loss of body heat while cushioning vital organs. People with high blood triglyceride levels tend to have low

HDL (good) cholesterol levels. That's bad news for type 2 diabetics for two reasons, because it makes them vulnerable to atherosclerosis and because as obese people run out of normal fat storage space, the triglyceride molecules invade tissues where fat does not belong and this interferes with normal organ function.

There are two sources of triglycerides. You can eat them in the form of animal fat and some plant fats (like palm oil) or your body, specifically your liver, can make them. When eaten, triglycerides are absorbed through the wall of the small intestine, and then transported as a liquid through a network of thousands of capillary-like tubes called lacteals. The lacteals merge as they ascend the abdomen and proceed alongside the aorta into the chest, where they coalesce to form one flimsy tube, the thoracic duct, which, in turn, passes under the clavicle and empties into the left jugular vein. From there the triglycerides flow, mixed with venous blood, to the liver. Surgeons can observe this process. Ordinarily we wait eight hours after our patient has eaten before operating. We want our patients' stomachs empty to avoid the possibility of vomiting while under anesthesia. Eight hours after eating the transparent lacteals are empty too. They're invisible. But occasionally an emergency finds us in the belly of someone who has just had a meal and their lacteals are filled with milky-white triglycerides. They stand out like thick, white spider webs on the bowel's surface. Only surgeons are privy to this view of physiology in action; no other physicians see it.

Arteries have many important functions. They are not simply pipes that carry oxygen-loaded blood from the heart to the tissues of the body. They play a large role in maintaining normal body temperature and proper organ function. Arteries have muscle in their walls, and a plexus of nerves enables them to dilate and contract. For example, the small arteries in the skin will contract when exposed to cold, and shunt warm blood to vital internal organs. Exposed to warmth, they dilate, lending a pink blush to the skin. It's the same trick desert rabbits and African elephants use to let body heat escape through thin-skinned ears. And, unlike simple pipes, if arteries are accidentally sliced in half, their muscular walls automatically contract like a sphincter to quickly stop the flow of blood, a handy natural defense against exsanguination in this era of land mines and improvised explosive devices. During wound healing, the arterioles, the smallest of the arteries, at the wound's edge dilate to increase oxygenation; this enhances the healing process. Most important, the thin-walled capillaries release oxygen to the tissues and take in carbon dioxide for transport to the lung to be exhaled. The disruption of all these blood vessel-mediated physiologic processes is a hallmark of longstanding diabetes.

In the diabetic or the smoker, obstruction of the arteries in the pelvis and legs impedes the delivery of oxygenated blood to the muscles used for walking. This is a painful condition. Typically, the patient with arterial obstruction in the legs is able to walk a short distance, but must stop periodically and rest until the pain subsides (until the leg muscle's oxygen supply is replenished). This phenomenon is called *intermittent claudication.* We measure severity of claudication in units of city blocks. Someone with mild claudication may be able to walk two blocks before he must stop and rest. He is "a 2-block claudicator." A severe claudicator may develop calf pain at half a block. The location of claudication pain depends upon the location of the arterial blockage. If the arteries of the pelvis or thigh are closed, the pain may appear in the buttocks or thigh, but in most diabetics the pain is in the calf. The more extensive the blockage, the more severe the claudication; the steeper the incline, the quicker the onset of the pain.

Claudication is the first symptom of impaired circulation to the legs, and smoking or the blood vessel-damaging effect of diabetes is the most likely cause. The best treatment for claudication, aside from the obvious — stopping smoking and treating the diabetes — is to walk — to walk until the pain appears, then rest until it goes away (a minute or two), then walk some more. Walking builds up *collateral circulation.* That is, it promotes enlargement of secondary blood vessels, nameless branches which compensate for the blocked artery by detouring blood flow around it. The worst mistake a claudicator can make is to limit his walking; that enables the arteries to clog up faster. There are medications available to treat claudication; unfortunately they are expensive and often ineffective.

Diseased arteries are a challenge to fix. The risk of surgical complications is real. So arterial bypass surgery or arterial stenting should never be an elective or incidental procedure. Ethical surgeons, invasive cardiologists, and radiologists perform these procedures only for patients whose claudication is incapacitating, whose leg pain occurs when simply walking from room to room, or for those who have pain at rest, or a non-healing wound due to lack of blood flow. Operations, angioplasties, and stents should never be done to assure a pain-free round of golf, or relieve one block claudication. But we have a market medical system; doctors get paid for what they do, and hospitals profit from procedures, so beware of the "drive-by angioplasty" — one done during the course of a diagnostic arteriogram or a cardiac catheterization, when the angiographer (it may be a surgeon, radiologist, or invasive cardiologist) comes across an *asymptomatic* narrowing in a major artery, one that is not related to the procedure at hand, and is tempted and then proceeds — in spite of the risks — to stent that artery on the spot.

Diabetes and Cigarettes

In his 1938 short story, "The Secret Life of Walter Mitty," James Thurber's hero is a man consumed by daydreaming. Walter's mind wanders to escape a banal life with a domineering wife. In one daydream, he is a world-renowned surgeon summoned to the operating room to help two other famous surgeons. They're operating on an "important patient" with an acute abdominal condition. They open the abdomen, they look around, and they find it's too late — "Coreopsis has set in." Coreopsis, of course, is not a disease, it's a plant species. I think of this imaginary circumstance when I encounter a very real "too late" situation, not "coreopsis," but non-remediable arterial obstruction from cigarette smoking. A diabetic patient who smokes will often develop a too-late-to-fix situation — advanced arterial occlusive disease. One in twenty smokers will get lung cancer, but more often, longterm smokers develop limb-threatening peripheral artery disease. Smokers and diabetics are the bread and butter of any vascular surgery practice. They develop arterial blockage that may involve the coronary arteries in the heart, the arteries of the kidneys, the carotid arteries in the neck, or the blood vessels of the eye. But most frequently it's clogging of the arteries of the legs and feet that initiate a trip to the vascular surgeon's office.

The most common cause for hospitalization of the diabetic patient is a foot problem.[2] Diabetic foot problems are caused and compounded by poor circulation, neuropathy, and pressure on bony prominences. Our hospital has a 30-bed diabetic unit, but many more diabetics fill beds throughout the hospital. More than half the patients in those beds have a limb-threatening foot problem. I couldn't count the number of feet I've been called upon to salvage. The most commonly encountered diabetic foot afflictions are depicted in figure 3. Aside from obvious coexisting health problems, I never connected a patient's infected foot to his general health. But diabetic foot infections, it has been proven, often precede more serious health problems.[3] Recent studies indicate that almost half of these patients will eventually undergo an amputation, and, alarmingly, within six and a half years after hospitalization for a foot problem, more than half of these patients will have died.

Here is a list of the most common diabetic foot problems:

• Trophic ulceration occurs most frequently on the ball of the foot where pressure on numb skin from the misaligned, bony ends of the metatarsal bones goes unnoticed because of neuropathy. Ulceration can be avoided with soft leather, form-fitted shoes. But once an ulceration forms, surgical removal of the metatarsal head is often required.

• Dry gangrene of a toe is the result of occlusion of both digital arteries (each toe is nourished by a pair of arteries). These small, calcified vessels may fracture and clot, so dry gangrene of a toe may appear even when leg circulation is adequate.

• Fissures are cracks in the skin, usually on the heel; they result from dry skin where sweat glands have been destroyed by neuropathy. They can be painful even if the circulation is good, or painless if neuropathy is severe. The prevention is daily application (in small amounts) of cocoa butter or lanolin-based moisturizers.

• Pressure sores (Decubitus ulcers or bed sores) occur most frequently on the heel, are preceded by redness, and can be prevented, in bedridden patients, by placing rolled towels under the ankles and applying Velcro secured heel pads. Pressure sores may be blamed on poor nursing, but ultimately are the fault of any unobservant doctor, resident, or nursing aide — anyone involved with the patient's care.

Note that all of these diabetic wounds occur below the ankle. Wounds above the ankle are most often due to vein problems, chronic venous stasis ulceration. Diabetics, particularly overweight diabetics, are plagued with these as well. My treatment is elevation of the foot of the bed if the circulation is adequate, debredement when dead tissue is present, and the wet-to-dry dressing technique (see wound care, page XXX). Venous stasis leg ulcerations heal extremely slowly.

Peripheral Artery Disease: The Case of Annie Walker

Why are foot problems so prevalent in diabetes? Remember Annie Walker? We met her on her way to the operating room. She was diagnosed with type 2 diabetes while in her late 30s. Since then, she contends, she's taken good care of herself. She changed her diet, joined a gym, and lost some weight. Nevertheless, over 19 years, she progressed from diet control,

The Common Diabetic Foot Problems

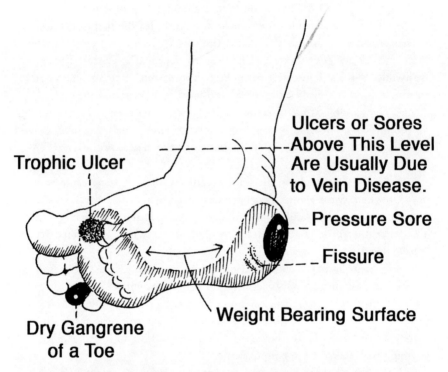

Ulcers or Sores
Above This Level
Are Usually Due
to Vein Disease.

Trophic Ulcer

Pressure Sore

Fissure

Dry Gangrene
of a Toe

Weight Bearing Surface

Fig. #3: Common diabetic foot problems. Foot problems are the leading cause for hospitalization of the diabetic. *Trophic ulceration* occurs most frequently on the ball of the foot where pressure on numb skin from the misaligned, bony ends of the metatarsal bones goes unnoticed because of neuropathy. Ulceration can be avoided with soft leather, form-fitted shoes. But once an ulceration forms, surgical removal of the metatarsal head is often required. *Dry gangrene of a toe* is the result of occlusion of both digital arteries (each toe is nourished by a pair of arteries). These small, calcified vessels may fracture and clot, so dry gangrene of a toe may appear even when major leg circulation is adequate. *Fissures* are cracks in the skin, usually on the heel; they result from dry skin where sweat glands have been destroyed by neuropathy. They can be painful even if the circulation is good, or painless if neuropathy is severe. The prevention is daily application (in small amounts) of cocoa butter or lanolin-based moisturizers. *Pressure sores* (Decubitus ulcers or bed sores) occur most frequently on the heel, are preceded by redness, and can be prevented, in bedridden patients, by placing rolled towels under the ankles and applying Velcro-secured heel pads. Pressure sores may be blamed on poor nursing, but ultimately are the fault of unobservant doctors, residents, nursing aides, or anyone involved with the patient's care.

to pills, to self-injected insulin. She's still slightly overweight and still smokes. And smoking, we know, causes rampant arteriosclerosis in the diabetic.

Annie's problems began simply enough. On the Monday before I saw her she went to a school board meeting wearing her new, pointy, red shoes. That was enough for a diabetic, one whose nerves don't work and whose arteries are blocked, to get caught in a cascade of dire consequences. From the start, she felt no pain from the bruise on the ball of her foot. But the following Thursday, she saw a stain on her stocking and, using a mirror, she found the problem, a broken blister. No big deal, she thought. She washed the wound, slapped on a plastic patch bandage, and started wearing sneakers. By Tuesday, it looked worse; the foot was a little swollen. She had to leave that sneaker unlaced. By Wednesday, she had a fever. She called a podiatrist. He saw her that day. As he removed the bandage, he looked up and explained that sealing her sore with a plastic patch was, in effect, creating a little greenhouse, an incubator for bacteria. It's better to use simple gauze.

His first instinct was to check her circulation. He felt for a pulse in both places on her foot where the artery should bound, but he felt nothing. Then he asked her to lie flat on her back, slid a chair to the foot of the examining table, slipped on some sterile gloves and, with a forceps and small scissors, removed the cap of dead skin. A few drops of yellow pus rolled from a shallow, dime-sized crater. He took a culture and sent it off to the lab. Then he covered the wound with a dime-sized disc of wet gauze, wrapped the foot with a gauze roll, and held it all in place with reusable elastic netting, no tape. He called Annie's husband in and explained that her circulation needed to be checked. He gave her a prescription for a broad spectrum antibiotic and, while the Walkers talked, he phoned me. He described what he'd done, and then, as if exposing a sin, whispered, "She's a smoker."

"Send her over," I said. "I'll squeeze her in."

Continuous flow of oxygenated blood is the key to wound healing, and vascular surgeons are, in effect, oxygen delivery men. When a wound's blood supply is blocked, too little oxygen nourishes it, so it will not heal. It will not heal, no matter what salves, ointments or potions are applied. The vascular surgeon's job, my job, is to determine if the blood supply is adequate, and if it's not — to fix it.

Annie's husband dropped her at my office door. Then, perhaps late for work, he disappeared. I happened to glance through the glass partition of Gail's reception area as Mrs. Walker limped up to register. Four patients sat waiting. They had a total of five legs among them. As luck would have it, none of them wore a leg prosthesis. Two were fresh post-ops and not fully healed, and the other two had stump problems, so they all used crutches. One fellow's new leg stood erect beside his chair, his hat propped on top. This was Annie's introduction to the world of diabetic complications. It was as if she'd walked in on a convenience store heist, and the take was legs. She stood there, trying not to look. How could she know that some of them started off just like her, with a trivial wound on the sole of their foot — one that would have easily healed were there no such thing as diabetes.

Gail took Annie's insurance information and sat her down. When I finished seeing my last scheduled patient, she led Annie to my examining room. The waiting room was empty now. On any other day there might have been one amputee, maybe none. Bad timing. I introduced myself and explained the purpose of her visit — to check her blood supply to see if it was it good enough to let her wound heal.

She was a well-padded, red-headed woman, smartly dressed except for the sneakers. Her black patent leather belt, cinched three notches beyond a worn groove, said she'd begun to lose weight. She fiddled with the strap on her purse, while behind her red-rimmed glasses her anxious eyes darted about the room. When she looked up, we saw that a large, crimson blotch had bloomed and begun to spread across the base of her neck. Gail gave her a reassuring smile.

We went through her history: 55 years old, married, no kids, no diabetes in the family. She'd worked several years as a teacher's aide, then returned to school and earned a teaching degree. Now she'd missed two days of work. She said she had no pain and the foot had only just begun to swell. The lack of pain was nice, I told her, but not normal. I asked if she knew what neuropathy was. She did. For years, she said, she'd had a tingling sensation in her feet, and sometimes, at night, even the touch of the bed sheets bothered her. Long ago she noticed that her feet were numb. She recounted her 19 years of diabetes and her gradual progression from diet to pills to insulin.

The phone interrupted us. I excused myself and went to my consultation room to take the call. Gail gave her a pink paper gown and drew the changing-nook curtain. When I returned, Annie was sitting on the edge of the examining table, transformed now from a proper schoolteacher to an ageing patient. Her glasses seemed thicker. Her hands were old. The pale skin of her neck and arms was loose; it drooped a bit, as if she'd worn a size too large. The crimson blotch, a not-so-subtle sign of apprehension, had spread across her chest. She looked down at her bare feet and casually asked how long it would take to heal. I hadn't examined her yet, but I knew then that she saw a bump in the road where I saw a land mine.

The answer flashed through my brain. I'd treated hundreds of diabetics with the same type of wound in the same place. So I knew that if her leg circulation was adequate, then with proper care it should heal in a week, maybe two. And if her blood supply was poor, then a surgical bypass or peripheral angioplasty would be needed. But if her blood supply were damaged beyond repair, then her seemingly simple sore would surely progress. The outcome would be unpleasant. I answered simply, "That depends on your blood supply."

I asked if walking caused her pain. Did she know the meaning of the term *claudication?* She could manage two blocks, she said, but then her right calf would tightened up — she'd rest for a minute or two, then go another two blocks. "It's worse," she said, "if I go uphill."

"How long have you been claudicating?" I asked.

"About a year," she said.

Claudication is the first sign of impaired circulation to the legs. As arteries fill with plaque, the claudication turns to pain at rest, or, in Annie's case, to a wound that will not heal (caused, for example, by tight, red, high-heel shoes). I didn't mention the third, unfixable, stage of arterial obstruction — gangrene.

From time to time I see patients who complain of severe cramping in the calf muscles. It awakens them at night. *Night cramps.* Many fear they have a circulation problem, but they don't. The cramps are due to abnormal quantities of calcium or potassium in the blood which throw the calf muscles into painful spasm; night cramps have nothing to do with circulation. They can be relieved by standing and stretching the calf muscle, or by pulling the foot back towards the knee. An old remedy is quinine, but it rarely works.

She pointed to her right foot, the one with the problem. It was red, while the left foot was pale pink. "Why the difference in color?" she asked.

"When the blood supply is poor," I explained, "and the foot hangs down, the skin capillaries dilate to compensate for the lack of oxygen. The rosy color gives the illusion of good circulation. It's a phenomenon called reactive hyperemia." I took the pulse in her wrist; 88 per minute, slightly fast. The nervousness, I thought. Her blood pressure was 160/85. The top number, the systolic, represents the pressure as the heart is pumping. The bottom number, the diastolic, represents the pressure in her arteries while the heart relaxes, as it refills between pumps.

There are many causes for high blood pressure. But diabetics tend to calcify their blood vessels, one reason why the top number, the systolic blood pressure, may be elevated. A systolic blood pressure of 160 millimeters of mercury was too high for Annie; her diastolic pressure, 85 millimeters of mercury, was acceptable. Hypertension (high blood pressure) is defined as a systolic over 140 or a diastolic blood pressure over 90. If left untreated, high blood pressure can lead to heart attack, stroke, and kidney failure. Hypertension is common in diabetics, especially in type 2s, and should be treated with weight loss when necessary and blood pressure medication. There's no effective treatment for the calcium in the walls.

Atherosclerosis is a patchy disease so, in the office, we check what we can, all the accessible arteries. The carotids are two of the four arteries that supply blood to the brain. The other two, the vertebrals, are in the back of the neck, encased in bone, and not accessible to physical examination. I held my stethoscope on Annie's neck, slightly below the angle of her jaw, and listened to her carotids; first the left, then the right. I explained that if her carotid arteries were narrowed by atherosclerosis, then blood passing through the narrow segment would speed up. The rapid blood flow through a narrowed artery causes a whistling or rumbling sound: a *bruit*, French for "noise." The presence of a bruit indicates partially blocked flow to the brain; it signals the risk for a stroke and demands further investigation, a carotid ultrasound exam. Her carotid arteries were silent; she had no bruit, no evidence of carotid artery disease.

I looked at her feet. She had cocked-up toes, a typical diabetic foot deformity. The clawed toes made her walk on the balls of her feet. With her diminished pain sensation and the wrong shoes, she was a setup for that foot wound. I peeled off the podiatrist's dressing and examined the sore. It was just as he said, a dime-sized, punched-out ulceration that sat directly over the ball of her great toe. He'd removed most of the dead tissue, but what remained was gray and spongy. It smelled of dead flesh, like a mouse kept too long in the trap. I used a sterile metal probe to see if the ulceration penetrated to the first metatarsal, the long bone in the foot that joins the first bone in the great toe. An ulcer that deep would suggest the presence of osteomyelitis, a bone infection. The probe stopped short of the bone. "Did you feel that?" I asked.

"No!"

Then I tickled the sole of her foot with my gloved index finger. "Did you feel that?"

"Yes!" She smiled.

Typically, a patient with neuropathy can feel touch, but not pain. The nervous system, I told her, is arranged in such a way that the sensations of pain, heat, cold, position sense, and touch each emanate from different receptors in the skin, specialized nerve endings, which connect to the various centers in the spinal cord and brain. If the pain receptors are knocked out, as in diabetic sensory neuropathy, then pain sensation is lost, but touch sensation remains intact. She could feel the stroke of a feather, but not pebble in her shoe.

The first sign of neuropathy is loss of position sense (proprioception). To test for it, I held Annie's big toe between two fingers and asked her to close her eyes. I moved the toe up, then down and asked if she knew what position it was in. She couldn't say; her neuropathy had erased her position sense, no surprise.

Diabetics can develop such numb feet that giving a surgical anesthetic, general, local, or regional, is unnecessary. It has only risks; no benefit. So complete is the sensory loss that toes can be removed painlessly, without anesthesia. Unfortunately, many surgeons don't realize this. All that's needed is a touch of sedation to take the edge off, and a cloth drape to block the patient's view. When the numbness is profound, the entire forefoot can be amputated painlessly, without anesthesia. Although the patient feels no pain from the prick of a pin or the slice of the scalpel, she may recoil from the touch of soft gauze; the receptors for touch are the last to go. Of course the patient can still hear, so I ask the anesthesiologist to turn up the volume of his music. That drowns out the crunch of metatarsal bones being cut. But that only works with older anesthesiologists; the young ones have iPods.

I listened to her heart — no murmurs, regular rhythm. I felt her abdomen, looking for signs of a palpable pulsatile mass, an aortic aneurysm. None was present. I palpated her femoral arteries. They're located just below each groin crease. Both were strong. Working my way down, I felt for the pulses in her popliteal arteries behind each knee. The left was okay, but the right was absent. Next, I placed my fingers on the dorsalis pedis pulses on the top of each foot. The left was present but weak. The right was gone, the artery blocked. I felt for the posterior tibial pulse on the inner aspect of the ankle; it's just behind the bony prominence above the instep (the malleolus). Nothing — no posterior tibial pulse could be felt in either foot. Her calf muscles were small and soft, atrophied from years of diminished blood flow. The skin on her legs was shiny, without hair stubble. No need for her to shave her legs; her circulation wasn't strong enough to nourish hair growth.

I carried my portable Doppler machine to the examining table. I wanted to more accurately assess the blood flow in her legs, particularly in those areas where I could feel no pulse. Doppler, or ultrasound devices (same thing), are used in various fields of medicine. In vascular surgery, we use them to listen to, or actually view, the blood flow in an artery or vein. In some cases it's helpful to gather technical information, like the velocity of the blood flow, the waveforms of the pulses, and the direction of the blood flow. By using blood pressure cuffs along with my Doppler probe, I can measure the pressure within a blood vessel at various levels in the leg. This helps me pinpoint the location of the blockage in an artery.

Human anatomy is consistent. The blood supply of a healthy leg arrives through one major vessel, the common femoral artery. This artery splits, or bifurcates, just below the groin. One branch, the profunda femoral or deep femoral artery, supplies the tissues of the thigh, while the other larger branch, the superficial femoral artery, continues down to the knee where it becomes the popliteal artery. There it branches again, into three smaller or medium sized arteries that supply the lower leg and foot. The two most important are the anterior tibial and the posterior tibial arteries. The third branch, the peroneal artery, peters out at about ankle level (figs. 4, 5).

I always Doppler the good leg first. That way the patient can hear and recognize the decreased or total absence of sound in the symptomatic leg. I wrapped the blood pressure cuff around Annie's left calf and held my Doppler probe on the top of her foot over the dorsalis pedis artery. I could feel the pulse there, under the probe. I inflated the cuff around her calf, then watched the mercury column fall as I let out the air — 200, 180, 150. When the manometer read 110 mm of mercury, the ultrasound machine began to wheeze the intermittent sound of the pulsating blood. At that pressure, 110 mmHg, the cuff was loose enough to allow blood to flow through the artery. I knew that with a Doppler pressure of 110 mm of mercury, she had adequate, not normal, but adequate, blood supply to her left foot. I placed my Doppler probe over the posterior tibial, the other artery in the left foot, and I repeated the process. The pressure there was 80 mm of mercury.

I moved to the right foot, the one with the problem. I put my hand under her heel, raised her leg to a level of 45° and watched the rosy pink

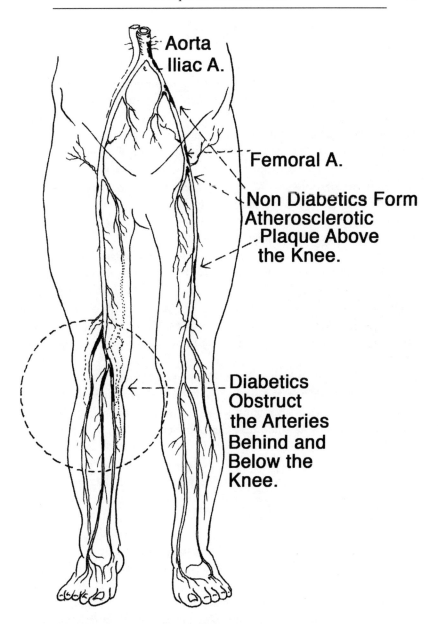

Aorta
Iliac A.

Femoral A.

Non Diabetics Form Atherosclerotic Plaque Above the Knee.

Diabetics Obstruct the Arteries Behind and Below the Knee.

Fig. #4: Pattern of arterial obstruction in the diabetic leg. Diabetics tend to obstruct the medium sized arteries behind the knee, the popliteal (anterior tibial, posterior tibial, and peroneal), whereas non-diabetics develop atherosclerosis and block the larger arteries of the abdomen (aorta) and groin (common femoral) and thigh (superficial femoral).

foot fade to white, a sure sign of blocked arteries. I put her leg down and began my Doppler examination. I knew the pressures would be lower in this leg, and they were. Instead of a loud, crisp Doppler sound we heard the faint swishing of meager blood flow. She looked down at her foot. I looked at her neck; the nervous red blotch had spread across her chest.

In the dorsalis pedis artery, the sound appeared at a pressure of 60 mm of mercury, and at 50 mm of mercury in the posterior tibial artery. The blood pressure in her arm was 160 mm of mercury, but the blood pressure in her right foot was only 50 to 60 mm of mercury. I repeated the process in her right thigh. The pressure there was 140 mm of mercury. My Doppler exam proved that Annie had a major arterial blockage somewhere between her thigh and her foot. I suspected the typical diabetic pattern, blockage of the medium-sized blood vessels behind the knee. Elderly non-diabetics and smokers, on the other hand, develop arterial obstructive disease in the larger arteries, the ones above the knee or in the pelvis (fig. 4).

I wiped the Doppler jelly from Annie's foot, helped her off the examining table, and asked her to come into my consultation room when she was dressed. I knew at that point she needed surgery to increase the blood supply of her foot. Without it, the wound would worsen; her leg was in trouble.

Annie's husband hadn't returned. She was alone. I offered to wait. "No." she said, "It may be a while." Gail knew the routine; she took the seat beside the patient. Annie understood now that she had a major circulation problem. She could hear the Doppler signal — loud in the good foot, barely a whisper in the ulcerated foot. She realized too, that even without pain, she had a problem. I explained that in order to heal, her blood flow had to be increased. Surgically increased.

I needed more information, the exact configuration of her arterial blockage. Only then could I give her the treatment options. My ultrasound examination was useful as a screening technique, but not detailed enough to use as a roadmap for arterial reconstruction. There are three basic methods of mapping arterial obstructions in the leg. The first is duplex imaging ultrasound examination, but it, too, is not detailed enough to see the medium and small vessel disease of the diabetic.

The second noninvasive option for evaluating the circulation is the MRA, magnetic resonance angiography. Although this test is noninvasive, it has its drawbacks. The patient must lie motionless on a hard X-ray table a long time, and, at this point in the evolution of medical technology, the test is not as good as standard arteriography, the third, oldest and most accurate method. Arteriography (or angiography) is done under local anesthesia; it's invasive. It's done by inserting a needle through the skin of the groin and directly into the femoral artery. Under X-ray guidance, a wire is then passed through the needle, and threaded up the artery. The needle is removed, leaving the wire in place. A hollow tipped catheter is then threaded over the wire and up the artery. The wire is withdrawn, leaving the catheter in place. Then radio-opaque dye is injected through the catheter, directly into the artery. Arteriography, therefore, comes with the infrequent, but very real risks of bleeding, damage to the artery wall at the puncture site, or embolization of plaque. (Particles of atheromatous material break off and lodge further down in the arterial branches causing damage to the toes. "Trash foot," we call it.) Rarely, an allergic reaction to the dye can cause anything from hives to anaphylactic shock. In diabetics, however, the major risk is chemically induced kidney damage, and with a nineteen-year history of diabetes, Annie's kidneys were a setup for trouble.

I explained the options and that if her kidney-function tests, her creatinine and blood urea nitrogen (BUN), were normal, then arteriography could be done and would give us the most accurate information. I explained that if, upon examining her, I had found evidence of blood vessel obstruction higher up, say in the groin or abdomen, then I would have suggested the MRA. But it was the blood vessels behind her knee that were her problem, and these smaller blood vessels can be evaluated best with arteriography. That gives us the most detailed picture. We needed an accurate roadmap so that we could plan the appropriate revascularization procedure, one that would deliver enough blood to her foot to assure healing and halt further damage.

I avoided the word amputation. No need to mention it. She should respond to some sort of revascularization procedure. She asked when we would do the tests. I told her I'd like to call her internist now, from the office. She'd need to have baseline blood work and an EKG prior to the arteriogram and I could expedite the appointment. I made it clear that the same process that was blocking the arteries of her legs, atherosclerosis, could be present in the coronary arteries in her heart. "No." she said. "I want to discuss it with my husband; I'll make the appointment."

"That's fine, but do it soon," I urged. "It's important that we get started on this." Her red-rimmed glasses magnified her eyes; they were fixed on the door. As she left with a tight-lipped smile I wondered, was I too emphatic? Was I not emphatic enough? Did I scare her off? Surgeons, they're too aggressive!

Four days went by; no word from Mrs. Walker. Then the E.R. called. It was 9 P.M. Annie's husband had taken her in two hours earlier. The E.R. physician described the foot. The ulcer was the size of a nickel now, and capped with a crusty scab. It had a nasty odor, he said. I requested a blood sugar, an EKG and the usual blood work, including kidney function tests. An hour later the E.R. physician called back with the results: the blood sugar was 340 mg percent (normal is 120); the white count was 16,400 (normal is up to 10,000). Her kidney function was normal, BUN was 30, slightly high, but she was dehydrated. Her serum creatinine, the true test of kidney function, was 1.4, the upper limit of normal.

The EKG showed an old, anterior wall myocardial infarct. Sometime in the past she'd had a heart attack. Annie was unaware of any heart problems, but silent, painless heart attacks happen in diabetics. Annie had never seen a cardiologist. I called the cardiologist on call for the day, Dr. Karen Woods. She arrived quickly, went over the EKG, and suggested that in view of the silent heart attack, Annie should undergo a stress test. That would detect any ongoing coronary artery disease.

I arrived just as the doctor was finishing her exam. I reminded her that Annie claudicated and couldn't tolerate a treadmill long enough to complete a stress test. She asked if we planned to do an arteriogram to evaluate her leg circulation, and if so, at the same time, could she evaluate the coronary arteries? In view of Annie's normal kidney function, I agreed to the dual procedure. We explained the plan to Annie and her husband. She would be admitted, started on IV antibiotics and, in the morning, be taken to the cardiac cath lab. Dr. Woods would do a cardiac catheterization and if Annie's coronary arteries were clear, then I'd pull the catheter down into the abdominal aorta, inject more dye and view the pattern of arterial obstruction. This, hopefully, would assure us that she wasn't about to suffer another heart attack. At the same time it would provide me with a roadmap for repair of the blocked artery in her leg.

Annie, shaken by the news of the silent heart attack, hesitated, but relieved to know it could all be done through one needle stick, she consented to the double procedure. I asked if her foot hurt. "No," she said. "It doesn't hurt." I took a look. Pus seeped from under the scab, hence the odor. It needed to be properly drained. Those of us who treat diabetic foot infections on a regular basis often can identify the major bacterial culprit (all diabetic foot infections contain multiple strains of bacteria mixed together) from the distinct smell and color of the pus. The pus oozing from Annie's foot was slightly green and had a nauseating, fruity, stench; the bacterium eating her foot was *Pseudomonas Aeruginosa.* I pulled on some sterile gloves, swabbed the area with Betadine and draped it off with sterile towels. I removed the scab. Creamy, greenish-white pus leaked out. I took a culture, irrigated with saline, and placed a new bandage.

It is so important to drain abscesses as soon as they are discovered. If left to drain by themselves, come to a head, they expand instead. They deepen towards the bone and track along the path of least resistance, usually up along the tendon sheaths. Valuable time is lost. We started Annie on IV antibiotics. She was given insulin to take her blood sugar down. And the cardiologist wrote orders in preparation for the cardiac catheterization. During the night, she was taken to a semi-private room on the diabetic unit. There the nurses would change her dressing every six hours and test her blood sugar every four. In the other bed, the one near the door, was an elderly, Spanish-speaking woman. She sat slouched forward. Her knees folded over the side of the bed, one hand gripped an IV pole, the other the edge of the mattress. One black shoe lay on the floor near the bed, the other, neatly laced, covered the end of a naked leg prosthesis, leaned against the closet door. She looked up and smiled.

Early the next morning Dr. Woods and I met Annie in the cardiac cath unit. The plan was to complete the cardiac phase, see the coronary arteries, and then pull the catheter down from the heart, position it in the aorta just below the renal arteries, and inject more dye in order to see the arteries of the right leg. It didn't work out that way. The coronary angiogram showed a 90 percent blockage of the left anterior descending coronary artery, the major blood supply to the left ventricle. Dr. Woods, anticipating the likelihood of finding such a problem, had obtained consent for possible stent placement. Finding the 90 percent narrowing, she did the prudent thing; she reopened the nearly closed vessel with a coronary artery stent. The problem was, to complete her work satisfactorily, she used the maximum quantity of contrast dye. Injecting more would likely damage Annie's kidneys. The leg study was canceled.

After the procedure, I found the Walkers in the cardiac cath lab. I explained that we still needed to study the blockage in her leg and suggested the next best test, an MRA. That would be noninvasive and require minimal dye, but it wouldn't be quite as accurate as an arteriogram. Also, it meant that Annie had to lie still on the X-ray table for 45 minutes. Claustrophobic people have trouble with that. Annie was nervous and suspicious, but she wasn't claustrophobic.

Noninvasive medical imaging procedures have become more and more accurate and, hopefully, will soon completely replace invasive diagnostic procedures. The MRA was done the next morning. It gave us a hard copy, and a dynamic picture of the arteries of her leg, groin, and foot. It confirmed my office findings. The main artery, the superficial femoral, was open with good blood flow, but further down, at the level of the knee, where the popliteal artery normally branches into three smaller vessels, there was obstructing plaque. Two of the three major branches, the anterior tibial and posterior tibial arteries, were closed. The third branch, the peroneal artery, which normally fizzles out below the calf, allowed only a trickle of blood to reach the ankle.

Annie's leg was severely oxygen deprived, ischemic. Ischemia is progressive. Mild ischemia causes claudication; moderate ischemia causes pain at rest, and severe ischemia leads to ulceration or gangrene. Ischemia from blocked coronary arteries causes heart pain, or angina. Annie felt fine; her neuropathy masked the pain.

As we suspected when we first examined her, Annie did have some collateral circulation; arterial blood flowing through enlarged branch arteries that originated above her blockage, coursed around that blockage, and then reentered her main artery. Collateral blood vessels form a natural detour, in effect a mini-bypass. Annie's collateral circulation helped keep her free of pain at rest, but wasn't developed enough to let her walk without pain or heal the wound on the ball of her foot.

Collateral blood vessels do not appear by chance. They form through purposeful walking on a regular basis; something Annie never did. Diabetics, indeed, anyone with blocked arteries in their legs, benefits from a strong or well-developed collateral blood supply. Strong collateral blood flow not only alleviates claudication and prevents rest pain; it can eliminate the need for leg bypass surgery, and act as a safeguard against amputation. Blood flow in the legs works on a use-it-or-lose-it basis. As time passes diabetics' arteries clog up. By establishing a walking routine early, preferably before any symptoms of claudication (leg cramps while walking) appear, diabetics can develop enough collateral blood flow to possibly avoid the surgeon (fig. 5).

For Annie's problem, blocked small and medium-sized arteries, the most effective treatment is a leg bypass using her own saphenous vein as the conduit. Veins have one-way valves, so after taking the vein from her thigh, it would be turned around so the bottom was the top and the valves reversed. Then it would be sewn into the artery above and below the blockage. This new channel would reestablish adequate oxygenated blood flow to her foot,

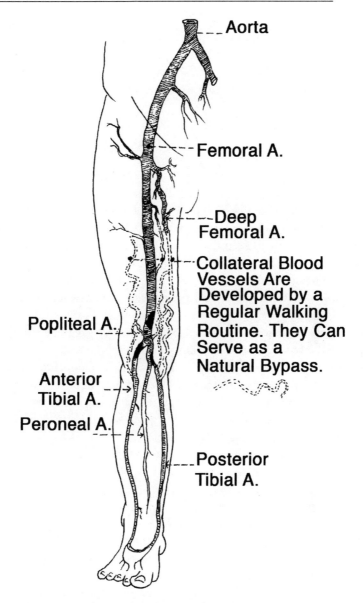

Aorta

Femoral A.

Deep
Femoral A.

Collateral Blood
Vessels Are
Developed by a
Regular Walking
Routine. They Can
Serve as a
Natural Bypass.

Popliteal A.

Anterior
Tibial A.

Peroneal A.

Posterior
Tibial A.

Fig. #5: Collateral circulation saves legs. Collateral circulation refers to the exercise-induced enlargement of small, nameless branch arteries which, by shunting blood around large blocked arteries, serve as a natural bypass to decrease claudication, eliminate rest pain, and, in some cases, safeguarding against amputation. Collateral circulation is developed through a purposeful walking routine.

allow the wound to heal, and eliminate her claudication. Without such a procedure, her infection would progress into the bone, travel along the tendons, and spread up the leg. Amputation would be inevitable. At this stage, antibiotics would do little; open arteries are required for delivery of the antibiotic to the infected area and Annie's arteries were closed.

Gangrene

There are two types of gangrene, *wet* and *dry*. Wet gangrene is dead tissue combined with infection. Dry gangrene is simply dead tissue, mummified, with no infection present. Wet gangrene cannot be cured with antibiotics; it rapidly progresses to sepsis, a bloodstream infection. We use antibiotics simply to keep the process from spreading. Dry gangrene cannot be helped with antibiotics either. Dead is dead. On the other hand, dry gangrene is not an emergency, though it should be treated before it progresses. If Annie had had dry gangrene, treatment would be less urgent.

Dry gangrene is not unusual in diabetics. It's the result of blocked digital arteries, the main arteries to the toes. Dry gangrene starts out as a purplish discoloration of the skin which, over the course of a few days, progresses to a coal-black mummified state. It's often painless in the diabetic with neuropathy. Gangrenous toes do not fall off as was once commonly believed. They must be surgically removed, preferably before the line of demarcation between the living and the dead tissue breaks down and provides an opening for infection.

As with any amputation, the surgeon must know, prior to operating, at what level the leg has enough blood supply to support healing. Just as in Annie's case, this requires adequate pre-operative assessment of the blood supply. In some cases, prior to doing the operation, an invasive diagnostic procedure is necessary. We want to keep as much of the limb possible, but a series of non-healing amputations, starting with the toe, then half the foot (transmetatarsal), then below the knee, then above the knee is the wrong way for the surgeon to proceed, and, needless to say, a great physical and psychological strain on the patient. The correct way to go about it is to study the blood supply beforehand and, when necessary, improve it with arterial bypass, stenting, or atherectomy. After that the surgeon can proceed with the amputation at the lowest level possible. It is essential to bring enough oxygenated arterial blood flow to the proposed amputation site before doing the amputation.

That evening, when Annie was back in her bed and the sedation had worn off, I went back to see her. Her nurse, Toni, was at the bedside testing her blood sugar. I greeted Mr. Walker and he introduced me to her cousin, Linda. Once again I explained that in order to save her foot, Annie would need an operation, a bypass graft. I sat on the edge of her bed, held the hard copies of the MRA up to the light, and pointed out the three blocked arteries, the cause of her festering foot. I outlined with my finger where the bypass graft would start, just above the blockage, and where it would be plugged into the open but nearly empty artery, the anterior tibial, in her lower calf. Her expressionless face conveyed reluctance. This would be a hard sell. I turned to Mr. Walker; he too was expressionless, apparently accustomed to her lack of trust. Finally he smiled and said, "That's great Annie; it can be fixed." All of us, Toni, Mr. Walker, the cousin and I awaited her consent, but instead we heard a plea for time — "At least the night," she said — to think it over. The cousin sat mute, eyes fixed on the roommate's prosthesis. Once again, I tried to reassure Annie, but the silence suggested I leave. They'd convince her. What choice did she have?

Annie had been through a lot in a week, and now she was facing major leg bypass surgery. Once again, her husband encouraged her to proceed, but once again she hesitated. She thought there must be an easier way. She hoped there was an easier way.

The following morning before rounds, the surgical residents, intern and I discussed amputations. In the United States, 1.2 million people live with amputations. More than half the amputees are diabetic. This figure, 1.2 million, refers to major leg amputations, above or below the knee. Toes are not included. The reason diabetics are so prone to amputation is their great propensity to develop accelerated arteriosclerosis. That tendency, together with an abnormal lack of sensation to pain (neuropathy), results in delayed diagnosis, impaired healing, and susceptibility to infection. Fortunately, many diabetic foot wounds can be successfully treated with proper wound care and, when necessary, revascularization procedures. So amputations can often be avoided.

There is always some initial trauma. A blister from a hike, a nick from a shell on the beach, a fissure in dry skin. It may appear to be minor, but it initiates the cascade of events that lead to amputation. Annie Walker blamed it on the new shoes, but it wasn't quite that simple. Longtime diabetics, especially those with neuropathy, often develop a specific type of foot deformity that predisposes them to trauma. Annie had that common foot deformity. She had cocked up toes.

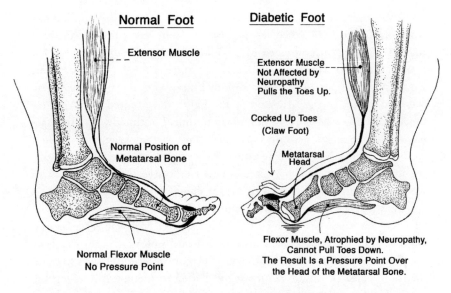

Figs. #6A and B: The most common diabetic foot deformity. The flexor muscles within the foot are weakened by diabetic neuropathy, but the extensor muscles, located above the ankle, are not affected by neuropathy. As a result of this imbalance, the toes are pulled up, "cocked," and the ends of the metatarsal bones are pushed down. Pressure is redistributed to the ball of the foot, where sensory neuropathy erases pain, and this makes this area vulnerable to ulceration.

In the normal foot, the toes project straight out. In the neuropathic diabetic foot, the toes become cocked up. They assume a cocked or clawed position because the muscles that pull the toes up are located in the lower leg, but the counterbalancing muscles, those which pull the toes down, are located in the foot itself. The nerves that control the muscles in the foot (the flexors) are easily damaged by motor neuropathy; they stop working. However, the nerves that control the muscles of the lower leg (the extensors) are not affected by motor neuropathy. Unopposed, they pull the toes up in a cocked position (fig. 6).

When you walk with cocked up toes, the pressure is redistributed to the ball the foot (the metatarsal heads). Excess pressure on the ball of the foot causes trauma to the skin, trauma that is not felt by the neuropathic diabetic. This type of foot trauma is so common in diabetics that it has its own name: trophic (resulting from interruption of nerve supply) ulceration. That's what happened to Annie. She put on her new shoes, but they did not accommodate her cocked up toes. She bruised the numb skin over the vulnerable heads of her metatarsal bones and developed a trophic ulcer on the ball of her foot.

How Wounds Heal

Frank, the intern who'd been following Annie's case, knew she was apprehensive. She was a quick healer, she'd told him. Surely she could find an alternative to going under the knife. The trouble is, there is no such thing as a quick healer. Healing takes two forms, each precisely choreographed and rarely off score. The physiology of healing has been defined on a cellular, biochemical, and molecular level; it is the same for everyone and is remarkably similar for all types of injured tissue — skin, muscle, bone, tendon, or fascia.

Which of the two types takes place depends upon the nature of the wound and the circumstances that caused it. Type one, called *healing by first intention* or primary wound healing, requires the assistance of a physician to bring the wound edges together. It takes place when there is no missing tissue between the two wound edges. Surgeons hope to see this type of healing with all their cases. The result is a nice, neat scar. The second type, *healing by second intention*, occurs when there is tissue loss or infection; for example, with open, traumatic wounds, infected lacerations (or surgical incisions), or deep burns, where a gap exists between the two edges. In 1888, when Van Gogh cut off his left earlobe in a fit of rage, his wound likely healed by second intent. This type of healing usually results in a prominent scar.

With first-intention healing the various tissue layers, muscle, fascia, and skin, are neatly sutured together; there is no gap. The process takes place step by step. First minor capillary bleeding ceases with clot formation (a complex cascade of biochemical events in its own right). Small arteries stop bleeding as the cut vessels constrict. This is followed, on the first day, by the inflammatory phase in which the blood vessels at the wound's edge become engorged, creating a blush or inflamed look. Inflammation (not to be confused with infection) is a natural part of the wound healing process and is confined to a centimeter or so around the wound edge. Inflammation beyond 2 or 3 cm signals the start of an infection. Next, white blood cells migrate to the cut edge to clear the dead tissue; they break down and engulf the damaged cells, a process called phagocytes.

At about 48 hours into the process, a glycoprotein called fibronectin begins to accumulate in the wound. It acts as body glue, holding the two sides together and confining the healing process to the wound edges. Fibronectin induces the growth of fibroblasts (new cells), fibrin, and collagen to gel together and connect one side of the wound to the other. Meanwhile, the injured cells at the wound edge spill various enzymes, histamine, prostaglandins, and platelet-derived growth factor (PDGF), into the wound. These substances initiate the process of epithelialization, the third phase of first intention wound healing. These enzymes stimulate the attraction of nearby epithelial (skin) cells, and cause them to reproduce and spread across the wound edges, fusing the two sides. Normally, epithelialization starts at 48 hours into the healing process and continues for about three weeks until healing is complete.

In the fourth and final phase, scar formation, PDGF causes fibroblasts (immature cells) to migrate to the wound edges and collagen bands to link across the wound. This strengthens the wound as time elapses. It takes only three weeks for skin to heal, but muscle, fascia, tendon and bone take months to complete the healing process.

Pharmaceutical companies have convinced consumers that vitamins, salves, supplements, and medicated bandages with enticing names can speed up the healing process. Unfortunately, there is no hard scientific proof that any of these products actually work. Undoubtedly, though, pseudoscientific entrepreneurs will continue to manufacture, advertise, and sell them, because pop culture validates them.

The healing process cannot be accelerated, but it can easily be slowed down. The major impediments to healing are infection, the use of steroids, very advanced age, kidney failure, and mechanical factors such as undue tension on the wound which pulls the edges apart. Walking on an open wound, say an ulceration on the ball the foot, will also impede healing.

Healing by Second Intention

Healing by second intention occurs with open wounds, wounds that are not sutured together. It takes place in three long phases. First there is the formation of granulation tissue, layers of cells that look like the surface of your tongue — red, wet, and granular. It has this appearance because it is rich in blood vessels, capillary buds, and fibroblasts, all of which replace the blood clot that appeared when the wound occurred. As with primary healing, white blood cells migrate into the wound from the surrounding normal tissue. They gobble up, or phagocytize, the dead cells, tissue debris and bacteria. Capillary buds develop and secrete enzymes, which break up the proteinaceous material, and fibroblasts migrate into the wound and produce collagen. The capillary buds evolve into small channels, blood vessels, which form a capillary network, enabling oxygen, white blood cells and nutrients to reach the area. The white blood cells engulf (phagocytize) and destroy the bacteria which inevitably blanket any open wound.

The richer the blood supply, the healthier (pinker) looking and more effective the granulation tissue in preventing colonization of bacteria (infection). Exposed white blood cells are short lived. When they die they remain on the surface of the wound as a thin white blanket of pus. That's what pus is — dead white blood cells. Pus, bacteria, and dead tissue debris can be removed easily with proper dressing change technique (described below). Relatively healthy patients with good blood supply, diabetic or not, will form a bed of granulation tissue over an open wound within a week of the injury — if that wound is kept moist. Once granulation tissue appears, then epithelial (skin) cells start to grow over it from the edges of the wound (epitheleization). The epithelial cells advance from all sides and eventually meet to close the wound.

While the wound granulates and as skin cells grow from the edges, a curious phenomenon takes place; the wound actually contracts. The open area shrinks like a drying puddle. The exact mechanism of this important aspect of the healing process, *wound contraction*, is not known. Most livestock farmers can tell you that healing in farm animals proceeds largely through wound contraction. If a goat or a horse sustains a six-inch laceration on its flank, within a week it will have contracted to three or four inches as it heals by secondary intention. The final stage of secondary wound healing is the exuberant accumulation of collagen, which gives these wounds a prominent scar.

Annie's open wound would have healed by secondary intention if she'd had adequate circulation. She would not have needed a bypass. A simple skin and soft tissue ulceration with no bone or tendon involvement and normal blood flow will heal with proper wound care. I would have simply debreded her wound, that is, removed the dead tissue, and started her on wet to damp dressing changes (the technique is described below), a very effective means of keeping a wound clean and free of surface bacteria. In addition, she would have been instructed to elevate the foot of her bed at night. Foot elevation is helpful only when there is adequate circulation to the legs. If leg circulation is poor, the feet ischemic, then elevation will decrease blood flow and cause pain. Foot elevation is best accomplished by placing paving blocks or books under the foot of the bed. That way the entire bed slants downward toward the head. Three or four inches are adequate. Placing a pillow or rolled up blanket under the foot never works. By morning, the pillow is usually on the floor.

Maggots, Miracles and Wound Care

Vijay, in his white dhoti and sandals, sat cross-legged like a Budda on a rug in Calcutta's steamy outdoor market. He spent his days selling fish. Victor, in his seersucker suit, sat in his swivel chair with his feet beneath a solid-oak desk. He spent his days selling stocks and bonds from his air-conditioned New York office on the 35th floor. Unlikely as it seems, Vijay and Victor had a lot in common: both men were fifty-seven, both were five feet nine, and both had type 2 diabetes—and more than that, each had a festering diabetic foot wound. Vijay's sore was between his first and second toes where the thong of his sandal wedged against his tender skin. Victor's was over the bunion where his black leather shoe pinched the protruding joint. Both men sought care of a specialist. Vijay went to the clinic at the Calcutta (Calcutta is now called Kolkata) City Diabetes Hospital (in India, where diabetes thrives, some hospitals treat only diabetics). Victor went to the high-tech wound care center in the University Hospital near his office.

When Vijay pulled his foot up to examine the tender wound more closely, he became alarmed—he saw something move—something Dr. Gupta had seen many times—maggots. They were the progeny, no doubt, of the common house flies that infested the marketplace. The doctor felt Vijay's foot pulses. They were strong and bounding. That alone proved that Vijay's blood flow was good. Then the doctor wedged a piece of clean white gauze between the sandal thong and the wound. He did not disturb the munching maggots; he left them there to their work. He knew they would clean the wound faster and more efficiently than any salve or surgical procedure he could provide. The doctor smiled and asked Vijay to return every four days for a dressing change.

Back in New York, Victor's wound care doctor took a long look and shook his head. First, quite properly, he felt Victor's foot pulses; they, too, were strong. Now the doctor knew that with proper care, his wound would heal. Then he asked the ultrasound technician to do a Doppler exam; he needed documentation. He swabbed the wound with antiseptic, injected some local anesthesia (which Victor did not need, as he had no feeling in the foot) and, using a scalpel and forceps picked away what dead tissue he could see. He prescribed an oral antibiotic (which Victor did not need), arranged for a dozen useless hyperbaric treatments (it costs a lot to run a wound center), two tubes of costly debriding ointment to be applied to the wound twice a day, and a week's supply of sterile gauze and elastic netting to hold the bandage in place. He arranged for a follow-up visit in a week.

After four weeks of maggot therapy (we actually call it *larval* therapy; it's less distressing) Vijay's wound was clean — that is, free of dead tissue — and new skin had started growing in from the normal skin edges. Dr. Grupta gently tweezed the maggots off and flushed them away. After four weeks Victor's wound was changed little. His doctor stopped the debriding ointment and, with his scalpel, again removed what dead tissue he could see. He prescribed a hydrogel absorbent pad dressing to protect the wound. He predicted that within a few months, with additional hyperbaric treatments, the wound should heal.

Though it seems absurd, these two cases are based in fact. Multiple well-conducted scientific studies as well as centuries of real life experience have proven, for the following reason, that maggots work better than conventional therapy for shortening healing time: they eat only dead tissue (they won't touch a healing cell) and they emit substances that kill bacteria (they are anti-microbial).[4] There are drawbacks, however; after forty-eight hours they can cause some pain or discomfort and, needless to say, they are not eye-pleasing.

All physicians hold one thing in common, a desire to cure or at least provide relief for our patients. I am not suggesting, with Vijay and Victor in mind, that we switch from conventional wound care to larval therapy (though maggots are commercially available). I am suggesting that physicians, and patients, too, have choices. There's more than one way to re-skin a cut. The average patient's choices are influenced by advertising on radio and television, the information provided on the internet, and the latest medical break-through. The physician's treatment plan hinges on a sound medical education, evidence-based success, and common sense — but sometimes our profit-based medical economy or the threat of a lawsuit (the medical chart is a legal document) gets in the way.

Wound Care Centers

Almost every large hospital in the United States has a wound center. These facilities might not exist were it not for the rising incidence of diabetes and its complications. Non-healing diabetic foot ulcerations are their bread and butter. Commercialism thrives in wound centers, making them a good source of revenue. Often, they are more proficient at healing a hospital's financial woes than a patient's open wound. Their effectiveness varies according to who staffs them, their choice of wound care products, and how ethical they are in their methods of treatment. The well-heeled hospital owns at least one hyperbaric oxygen chamber. Diabetic patients with open, nonhealing foot wounds are frequently subjected to multiple (20–40) costly ($200–$300/treatment) sessions in the hyperbaric chamber. True, all wounds require oxygen in order to heal, but they need it continuously. Oxygen delivered in short bursts, as in a hyperbaric chamber, provides no benefit in the healing of diabetic foot wounds. Years of observation have convinced me and other experts that hyperbaric treatments have no beneficial effect on wound healing in the diabetic foot.[5]

There are some good uses for the device. Hyperbaric chambers are, in fact, very effective in treating the bends, an excruciatingly painful condition that causes deep sea divers to double over in pain (thus the name). The condition is caused by the accumulation of nitrogen bubbles in the blood of deep sea divers who surface too fast. In a hyperbaric chamber, a short burst of high pressure oxygen drives the nitrogen from the bloodstream and reoxygenates the hemoglobin. But we see very few deep sea divers in our hospital. There is also some scientific evidence that the chambers aid healing in patients suffering from radiation burns. Diabetic patients, though, are wasting their money and time in hyperbaric oxygen chambers.

Enzymatic debreding ointments, salves that are intended to dissolve dead tissue, are expensive and, in my view, ineffective. However, they cause no harm (except to delay more effective treatment) and they do serve to keep the base of a wound moist, a necessity for wound healing. A well-trained vascular surgeon or podiatrist can clean up (debrede) a diabetic foot wound, that is remove the dead tissue, with a forceps and scalpel in a quick office visit, whereas the same ulcerated diabetic foot, treated in some hospital wound centers, may be subjected to weeks of fruitless and expensive hyperbaric chamber treatments, applications of ineffective salves or, even worse, harmful whirlpool soaks. Every wound seen in a wound care center heals by secondary intention.

The Care of Diabetic Foot Wounds

If the normal skin surrounding a diabetic foot ulcer is kept moist, it tends to macerate. If you've ever seen a floating swan, you may have noticed that they keep one leg up out of the water, adjacent to the wing. They let it air out, switching one for the other from time to time. They do this instinctively to prevent sores on their feet from maceration. The same goes for hard-shell turtles. They bask in the sun for two reasons. First, to increase their body heat and jumpstart their metabolism (they're cold-blooded), and second, to avoid tissue maceration and sores on their feet. Horses are no different. If left in a wet pasture day after day, they get foot rot. This is often accompanied by a fungal infection on the bottoms of their hooves. Constant moisture causes maceration (cell separation and skin-cell death) of human skin too.

Diabetics often lose sweat gland function in their feet because of neuropathy. They lose their natural skin emollients. This puts them at increased risk for skin maceration. The skin is the largest organ in the body. Its major function is to keep our body fluids from evaporating; it's the closed container, the wrapper that keeps us from drying up. Diabetic sensory neuropathy is essentially a foot-skin problem. Once the skin has broken down and a foot ulcer appears, meticulous wound care is required. The ulcer base (or ulcer bed) must be kept moist for healing to occur. At the same time, the surrounding skin must be kept dry to avoid maceration. Bacteria thrive in any ulcer bed or open wound, and bacterial growth impedes wound healing. If the wounds are simply bandaged and left for a day or two, then millions of bacteria build up on the surface and the healing process is impeded. Worse, if the patient were to place a plastic patch bandage over the wound, it would act as a small greenhouse and promote the growth of even more bacteria. Bandage companies know this, but cloth bandages are more expensive to make, so they make most with plastic. The same principle applies to scabs. Scabs are to be avoided with diabetic foot wounds, because, like plastic bandages, they trap bacteria beneath them, causing abscesses to form. Once again we can take a cue from the inborn habits of the animal kingdom. Most mammals instinctively lick their wounds in order to avoid scab formation and thereby prevent abscesses.

I have found the wet-to-damp method of wound care most effective (since maggots are taboo in our culture). In order to work, the wet-to-damp technique must be followed precisely. Here's the trick: cut the cloth

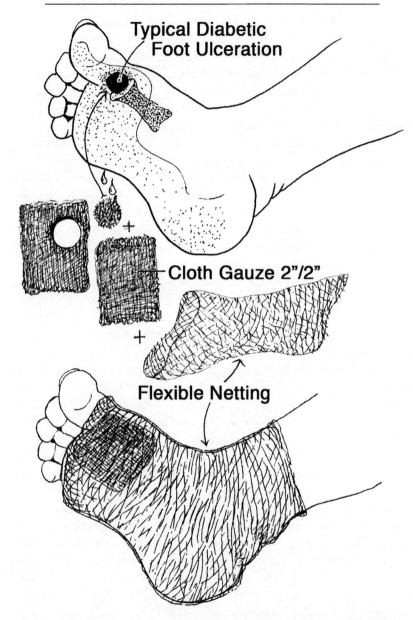

Typical Diabetic Foot Ulceration

Cloth Gauze 2"/2"

Flexible Netting

Fig. #7: Dressing change technique for diabetic foot and venous stasis ulceration. This method of wound care, like any wound care, only works if the arterial blood supply is adequate and in combination with surgical debredement (removal of dead tissue) when necessary. The details are described on page XXX.

gauze precisely to fit the open wound, wet it with clean tap or bottled water (sterile saline is not necessary) and place it in the ulcer bed. Take care to avoid overlapping the wet gauze onto the normal skin surrounding the ulcer. The normal skin around the ulcer must be kept dry, but the ulcer bed itself must be kept damp. By applying moist *cloth* gauze precisely cut to fit the wound, letting it partially dry over four to six hours, then peeling it off and replacing it with a new, precisely fitting, wet but not soaked gauze patch, the patient is both keeping the wound free of bacteria and protecting the tender cells at the base of the wound. The stage is set for healing. The bacteria and tissue debris adhere to the drying gauze and are discarded with each dressing change. Bacteria take about six hours to reproduce and start to colonize. By changing the damp gauze every four hours, infection is prevented. The process, somewhat akin to removing cat hairs from a couch with tape, keeps the wound clean, and the moist gauze acts like skin to keep tender healing cells from drying out.

It is essential that the normal skin around the wound be kept dry. With each dressing change, a dry 4 × 4-inch gauze pad is placed over the wet cloth gauze patch. No tape is used to hold it in place. Instead, tubular elastic netting, which can be purchased in any surgical supply store, is used to keep the bandage in place. Elastic wound netting looks like fishnet stockings; it was originally developed for burn patients. It has many advantages over tape, particularly when the dressing has to be changed several times a day. The netting stretches and can be purchased in the size appropriate for the part of the body part it needs to cover. (See fig. 7 for an illustration of this dressing change technique.) For me, this method of wound care has proven superior to any store-bought salve, ointment or patch. There is one problem though; *cloth* gauze is hard to find. Medical supply companies prefer to make cheaper 4 × 4 gauze pads out of *paper*. Paper gauze, when placed in a wound, leaves bits of paper debris. Paper gauze looks just like cloth, but you can distinguish it by ripping it. Cloth gauze can not be ripped. Fortunately, the 2 × 2 sized gauze pads are still made with cloth.

Annie Walker's Choice

When we'd finished our morning lecture and rounds, Sanjieve, the intern, and I went up to see Annie. We hoped to find her husband in her room and have her sign the surgical consent. I was looking to get her operated upon within 24 hours. Waiting longer would allow her foot infection to progress beyond repair.

The bed was empty. Annie was sitting in the bedside chair fully dressed, her red hair combed. She was ready to leave. Mr. Walker was standing, arms folded above his belt, staring through the window. He turned as we entered the room, shrugged, and said, "She's made up her mind," and he explained that during the night her cousin Linda had gone online. She'd found a nonsurgical alternative, a way for Annie to keep her foot and avoid surgery. There was a clinic, she learned, in New York State, where she'd be given injections that would dissolve the calcium in her blood vessels and open them up. "Chelation therapy," Annie said. And for the first time I saw a hint of a smile. Linda had Googled all the Web sites. There were so many! I sensed that she wondered why they weren't given this alternative. It was so common, so simple.

There were chelation clinics within driving distance, just over the New York State line. One of the Web sites said: "Now you can bypass bypass surgery!" Sanjieve and I looked at each other. We knew Annie had just gone through a battery of twenty-first century, state-of-the-art diagnostic and therapeutic procedures, procedures developed in the major scientific centers of the world, using the scientific method, taught in major medical schools and used with evidence-based effectiveness. Modern medical science had very likely saved her from a second heart attack and accurately identified her circulation problem, and now, if she could agree, would be used to restore the circulation to her foot and allow her to keep her leg. Instead, desperate to avoid surgery, hoping for a miracle, she turned to eighteenth century alchemy.

I knew nothing of Annie's roommate's history. The elderly woman, I assumed, had been admitted for dialysis treatments. I saw the bandages on her left arm. I caught a glimpse of her below-the-knee amputation stump. Her calf muscles were atrophied. The scar had healed years ago. Her prosthesis, which had apparently served her well, was practically an antique. All Annie saw was the fiberglass leg, like a piece of a mannequin, its black shoe for a foot, leaning against the closet door. She had to get out of there. She'd found hope on the Internet. Reason, it seems, can be hijacked by desperation.

Diabetics, indeed anyone, can fall victim to any number of schemes. They may be hatched from well-intentioned but misguided attempts to help, or from outright quackery. The uninformed diabetic may be duped by morally impaired entrepreneurs, economically driven wound centers, poorly trained physicians, or well-intended alternative healthcare practitioners pushing ineffective remedies like chromium for lowering blood sugar, hyperbaric chamber treatments, whirlpool baths or various ancient but "magical" concoctions of herbs to cure their diabetes or heal their wounds.

I took Annie's hand, looked her in the eye and told her she was making a mistake. It was as if she were leaving through the window, not the door. I wanted to rescue her. She looked silently at Mr. Walker. There was no changing her mind. I told her that hospital procedure required her to sign a form indicating that she was leaving against medical advice. She nodded. I walked with her husband to the nurse's station to get the form. He told me that Annie had trouble making decisions and when she arrived at one it was usually wrong. He went to get the car. Annie signed the consent. The ward clerk sent for a wheelchair. Later, I learned that they had driven directly to the chelation center in upstate New York.

Sanjieve and I took a break from rounds. We went to the cafeteria for a cup of tea. I asked if he knew anything about chelation therapy. He knew it was a chemical process in which an organic compound is used to bind metallic ions to itself. This forms a stable, inert compound, which is soluble in water. In theory, the calcium in Annie's arteries would become attached to the chelating agent, be pumped through the bloodstream and pass out in her urine. The theory is sound. In fact, it's the chemical principal responsible for the effectiveness of water softeners. Scientific studies done by the National Institutes of Health have proven, however, that it is not in the least effective as a treatment for arteriosclerotic vascular disease, where it would be used, supposedly, to leach the calcium from arteriosclerotic blood vessel walls.[6]

The therapy is administered intravenously using EDTA (ethylene diamine tetraacetic acid). This chelating agent is usually administered over several hours as a weekly or biweekly infusion. It's quite expensive. Because the treatment is not accepted as effective, or even ethical, by mainstream medicine, it is not covered by insurance. The patient pays out of pocket. And as a nonconventional or alternative form of medical treatment, there is no standard protocol for its administration. It varies from clinic to clinic. The technique of chelation therapy is not taught in medical schools, though it may be mentioned as an example of quackery. Accredited community and university hospitals do not offer it as a form of treatment for arteriosclerosis.

In spite of this, many freestanding chelation clinics continue to attract patients. They use anecdotal examples of its effectiveness while ignoring scientific proof that the chelating agent, EDTA, a water soluble substance, is incapable of attaching itself to the calcium in arterial walls. Fortunately, the infusion of EDTA has relatively few side effects. In Annie's case, though, the treatments provided time for wound bacteria to multiply and tissue to die. It placed her leg in jeopardy.

A Call to the E.R.

Annie's husband called on Saturday evening at 7 P.M. They were on their way back to the hospital. The foot didn't look good. He had seen enough. I called the E.R. and asked the triage nurse to draw a stat blood sugar and call me when Annie arrived. I got there at 9 P.M. This time I found her in bed 13, an isolation room. Dr. Lee was on call again. He had already received the blood sugar, 410; she was given insulin and was just back from X-ray. Dr. Lee wanted to check for gas bubbles in the tissues of her foot and leg. Severe infections, those caused by Streptococcus or Clostridium organisms, emit gas which spreads through the tissue planes under the skin and between the muscles. The gas shows up as black patches on an X-ray film. Gas-producing infections demand immediate surgical attention; they spread quickly. There was no gas. An examination, though, showed that the infection had entered the flexor tendon sheath of the great toe and burrowed deep into the plantar space in the sole of the foot. Tendon sheaths provide a path for bacteria to ascend into the lower calf. A faint red streak was visible in her skin. It extended from her ankle up the calf towards her groin. She'd developed lymphangitis. The lymph nodes in her right groin were palpably enlarged.

Ellen, her E.R. nurse, came to take vital signs and start an intravenous drip. She asked Annie how she felt. "Fine," she answered. Annie's temperature was 102 F. I asked Ellen to draw blood cultures.

"Do you know where you are, Annie?" I asked.

"Home," she said blankly.

Mr. Walker confirmed that she'd been confused all day. I told him that he'd have to be the decision-maker for now. A nurse's aide arrived with Annie's first dose of antibiotics and hung it on the IV pole. I asked Ellen about the bed situation. "No empty private beds in the hospital," she said. Then she turned to Mr. Walker. "We'll watch her here tonight," she assured him. "A bed should open up by morning." I called for Sanjieve; I wanted to show him how to drain an infection that had progressed into the tendon sheath. He was off again.

Mr. Walker signed the consent for me to drain the abscess. Ellen and I gathered the equipment: a scalpel, dressing set, peroxide, wound culture set, sterile gauze, and netting to hold the bandage in place. Ellen brought a 10 cc syringe and a vial of Xylocaine, a local anesthetic. I washed my hands. Then I drew the local anesthetic out of its ampoule, and exchanged the needle for a smaller one. I slipped on my sterile size 7½ gloves. Ellen lifted Annie's foot and propped it on a folded green sheet.

I asked Mr. Walker if he wanted to leave the room. We didn't want him fainting in the middle of this. "It's okay," he whispered. Then he turned his chair to avoid the scene. Somewhere between confused and inert, Annie lay staring at the ceiling. I said nothing. Why disturb her? I gently probed the soul of her puffy pink foot with my index finger; pus poured from the open wound at the base of the big toe. It continued to drip on the green towel as my finger marched towards her heel. I heard a gag from behind the curtain separating us from the next cubicle. The foul stench of dead tissue and pus had wafted through. Instinctively, I breathed through my mouth to avoid the odor. I picked up the needle-tipped syringe and, testing for pain sensation, pricked a little trail from the ulcer at the base of the big toe to her heel. No reaction.

I put the syringe down, picked up the scalpel, and made an incision through the full thickness of the skin from the ulcer to a point just short of the heel. Yellow pus poured out. As I started, Ellen grabbed the Xylocaine-filled syringe and blurted, "Aren't you going to..."

"Doesn't need it," I said. "She's neuropathic."

Annie didn't budge. The pus soaked through the towel. I irrigated the incision with peroxide, and gave the foot a gentle squeeze to be sure no pus remained. Then I packed the wound with saline-soaked gauze, wrapped it with a sterile bandage, and covered it with flexible netting. As we peeled off our gloves, Ellen remarked, "Strange. There was no bleeding."

"I know," I said. "That's the problem."

I completed the E.R. chart recounting Annie's brief history: the podiatrist, the first visit to my office, the first hospitalization, including the angioplasty and the findings on the MRA, and her misadventure with the chelation people. I noted her confusion, high blood sugar, and pending blood cultures. In order to document the extent of the infection, I drew a simple diagram of her foot showing the location of the infection and the extent of the drainage procedure (fig. 8a). I wrote admission orders, explained how to change the dressing every four hours, and requested that the foot of the bed be kept flat. I underlined "no sedation or pain medications." Annie was already confused; sedation would make it worse. Diabetic foot infections are always polymicrobial, meaning they are caused by multiple types of bacteria, so I started her on a broad spectrum intravenous antibiotic. I ordered that she take nothing by mouth (NPO), wrote IV fluid orders, and placed her on an insulin drip — 25,000 units of regular insulin in 250 cc of saline, administered by an intravenous pump and calibrated to keep her blood sugar in a range between 80 and 110 mg percent. This would require finger stick blood sugars every four hours. Anticipating the need for surgery in the morning, I wrote an order for the blood bank to type and cross her for two units of packed red blood cells. We probably wouldn't use it, but better to be prepared.

Annie was dozing when I returned to room 13. I motioned Mr. Walker out of the room, sat him down in the doctor's area and told him what he didn't want to hear. "How far up?" he asked, and then added with unmasked panic. "Tonight?"

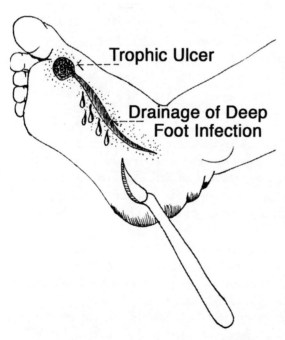

Trophic Ulcer

Drainage of Deep Foot Infection

Fig. #8a: Annie Walker's drainage procedure.

"No," I told him. "I'll reassess her on morning rounds. She'll be less toxic then and hopefully her confusion will have cleared." Imagine being taken to the O.R. while your brain is, in effect, on vacation, and then when it returns discovering that one of your legs is missing. Taking a confused patient to surgery is a hard choice for a surgeon, and except in dire circumstances, unfair to the patient. I explained that with the abscess drained, the fever should drop, and the insulin drip would stabilize her blood sugar.

"Tomorrow's Sunday," he said.

"I know; I'll be here at eight."

I left the E.R. and was halfway down the hall when I felt a tap on my shoulder. It was Dr. Lee. "Would you mind seeing the woman in bed 2?"

"You know," I said apologetically, "I'm not on E.R. call tonight..."

"I know," he said. "But it's late, and by the time I get Riley to come in," he was the general surgeon on E.R. call, "you know what happens. He'll call the resident, the resident will send the intern, he'll order a bunch of tests, and it'll be morning before anything's done."

"What's your problem?" I asked.

"An old lady with abdominal pain," he explained.

We walked back to bed 2. I opened the curtain and found a frail, gray-haired, elderly lady. Her bony right hand clutched a green plastic emesis basin. Her left was knotted to her daughter's, who sat in the bed-side chair. I introduced myself and asked the old woman what was bothering her.

She opened a toothless mouth, but it was the daughter who spoke. "She's got an awful stomachache. She hasn't eaten all day."

"I'm a surgeon." I said. "And your name is?"

"This is Ruth; I'm her daughter."

"Has she ever had pain like this before?" I asked, thinking the woman was mute.

"Yes, it's happened two or three times in the last couple of months, but it's never lasted this long, almost two hours."

I pulled the curtain closed; Dr. Lee wandered off, his responsibility dumped in my lap. "Let's take a look," I said. I drew the sheets down and peeled up her gown. Her belly was distended; the tense skin glistened like a beach ball. I heard bowel sounds even without using my stethoscope. She was thin, Halloween thin. I could see her femoral arteries pulsating in both groins, her blue veins through the translucent skin of her thighs, and her ribs heaving with each breath. In the left groin, just above the bounding femoral artery, was a walnut-sized lump. "Ruth, how long have you had this lump?" I asked.

"What lump?" the daughter responded. "This one, here in her groin," I said, as I gently kneaded it with my fingertips.

"She has a hernia, an incarcerated hernia," I said. "There's a loop of bowel stuck in it, and that's what's causing her abdominal pain. She's got an intestinal obstruction."

"Does she need an operation?" the daughter asked.

"I'm afraid so." I said. "But you say she's had the bellyache for how long, two hours?"

"Yes, about two hours," she said.

"Apparently with those other painful episodes the hernia reduced itself, so we'll try to reduce it here in the E.R. If the knuckle of bowel doesn't slip back into her abdomen within a few hours, she'll need to go to the O.R."

I tried to push the bulging knuckle of bowel back into her belly, to reduce the lump by pressing down with a gingerly massage. No dice. I asked if her mom was able to lie flat in the bed without having trouble breathing. This time, the old lady answered. "Sure," she said, "but I need a pillow." I adjusted her bed so that the foot-end was elevated several inches and the head sloped down, pulled an extra pillow from the linen cart beside her bed, and put it beneath her head. I told her I'd be right back, and went to the ice machine and filled a size 8 latex glove with ice chips. I put a washcloth over the lump and placed the cold lumpy glove on top of it. I taped it loosely in place. I called Ruth's nurse to the bed-side, showed her the ice pack, and asked if she'd check it every half hour. "If that lump disappears," I said, "remove the ice pack."

I told the old lady I'd return to check her in a few hours, filled out the chart, and canceled the CAT scan ($1,800) Dr. Lee had ordered in lieu of a thorough physical exam. I ordered the usual preoperative workup including a chest X-ray and EKG. Then I went to find Dr. Lee. He was at the nurses' station sipping coffee. I explained the findings and requested he keep her there, in the E.R., until I got back. I called the operating room desk clerk and requested that she add both Annie and the old lady to the A.M. surgical schedule. The old lady was not a diabetic. If she were, I would not have had the luxury of watching her for a few hours. Diabetics need prompt surgical attention. Their history and physical findings don't often correlate with the severity of their problems, and timely surgery will avoid complications.

I was out of the E.R. by midnight, slept without a call, and was back at 6:30 A.M. My first stop was the emergency room, bed 2. A different E.R. nurse was in with the old lady. She was hanging a new IV bag. The daughter was still in the chair, sleeping with her head rolled back and her mouth wide open. I touched her shoulder and said, "Good morning." She jerked her head forward, looked at her mother, then at me, and asked the time. "About twenty to seven," I said. "Let's have a look at that hernia."

I uncovered the old lady's belly, and removed the ice pack. The beach ball had deflated and the lump was gone. The cold pack had reduced the swelling and gravity, her head down and her feet up, had allowed the loop of bowel to slip back to its normal position. "How do you feel, dear?" I asked.

"Hungry."

I told her that we would repeat her blood work, get her a liquid breakfast, and observe her for a few hours. Then, after lunch, if she felt okay, I told the daughter, she could take her mother home. I gave her my office telephone number and explained that the hernia still needed to be repaired. "But now," I said, "we can do it as an outpatient procedure, under local anesthesia."

I called the O.R. and took her off the schedule. "Okay!" said the O.R. nurse. Nothing makes an O.R. nurse happier than a cancellation on Sunday.

"And what about the other case, Annie Walker?" she asked.

"I'm going up to see her now. I'll get back to you in 15 minutes." I wrote a note in the old lady's E.R. chart, then I headed up to the diabetic unit. The E.R. staff had transferred Annie there during the night.

I found Annie's nurse, Toni, on the diabetic unit. She told me Annie had had a pretty good night. Her temperature was down to 100.7, but she'd had some teeth-chattering chills. Her blood sugar was down to 120 mg percent, the insulin drip was at .8 units per hour, and she seemed alert. Her confusion had cleared with the rising sun. The night nurse had just changed the dressing. Mr. Walker, looking tired and apprehensive, stood outside her door. He hadn't mentioned the word "amputation" to Annie. "That's good." I told him. "That's my job."

Yes, she was alert. Her red hair was brushed and her glasses were down on her nose. She looked me in the eye as if to ask, "What's next?"

I asked her how she felt. Did her foot hurt? "I feel OK," she said. "My foot doesn't hurt." She had that embarrassed look some patients get when they know they've been disoriented and then regain their senses.

I told her I'd have to change the dressing even though it had just been changed. Toni and I pulled on some gloves, took down the bandage, and peered into the gaping wound. No blood, two exposed tendons, the head of the first metatarsal bone and some spongy, gray, dead tissue. The odor had diminished. Testing for residual pus, I placed my hand around her ankle and gave a gentle squeeze; no pus. The infection apparently hadn't yet traveled up the leg. Annie announced that she was ready for the bypass. Mr. Walker looked at me, and then at the floor.

I removed my gloves and sat down in the bedside chair. I explained that now, in the presence of such a severe infection, a bypass was no longer possible, and even if we attempted it, the exposed necrotic tendon and bone, in the long run, would lead to an amputation anyway. At that point my cell phone mercifully interrupted us. It was the microbiology lab. Annie's blood cultures had come back positive. They were growing MRSA, methacillin resistant Staph Aureus, a bacterium untreatable with the usual antibiotics. The bloodstream infection, septicemia, explained the teeth-chattering chills.

"You're not taking my leg off?"

At least it was a question, not an ultimatum.

"Mrs. Walker," I said, "I'd like to tell you that there was an alternative, but there isn't any. That's the only way to get you better. The infection has entered your bloodstream. That was the lab on the phone." Her eyes welled up. To speak would unleash the tears. At times like this, it seems the vocal cords are directly attached to the lachrymal glands. She removed her glasses, rubbed her eyes, and shook her red head from side to side.

"Let's get you an infectious disease consultation," I said, knowing I needed backup. "We'll cover all the bases." She shook her head up and down. Mr. Walker reinforced my words with a nod.

"I'll see who's available. Be back in a few minutes."

I called the infectious disease office. The answering service picked up, but before I could speak she put me on hold. It's automatic. Then she informed me that Dr. English was on call. I told her it was urgent and gave her Annie's name, her room number, and the diagnosis. I left my cell phone number. I told Annie I'd finish my rounds and then return. Hopefully, by then, she would have had her second opinion.

It took me an hour and a half to see my remaining nine patients. They were scattered about the hospital in two buildings, over seven floors. My cell phone rang again. It was Sue at the O.R. desk. "Well, are you ready? The list is growing."

"I need a few more minutes," I told her. If I'd said "hours," she would have put me at the end of the schedule, sometime that night. I didn't want to wait that long, and Annie shouldn't have to wait that long. We have twenty-six operating rooms, but on Sundays only three are staffed. It was almost 8:30 A.M. when I got back to Annie's room. Dr. English still hadn't arrived. I called Sue back. She said she couldn't hold the room any longer. I asked who was after me on the list. She reeled off six cases, including a day-killing craniotomy. I convinced her to put me in the second slot, following a laparoscopic gallbladder. That would give me two hours to work this thing out.

I called Dr. English directly. He answered from his car. He was on his way to the hospital. I asked if he wouldn't mind seeing Annie first. Then I went to the doctors section of the cafeteria for breakfast. A good cafeteria is essential for a surgeon; we're there for breakfast and lunch six or seven days a week, and sometimes dinner, too.

There were two older surgeons at the table. Riley, the general surgeon who was on call the previous night, and an orthopedist named Knight. They were griping about the surgical residents. The usual topic, how they never seem to be around and how the new residency training regulations seem to have undermined their attitude towards the profession. The rigorous, day-in, day-out surgical training programs are over, they lamented, and the profession has changed from a lifestyle to a job. Of course, the new work rules were designed to assure that the house staff, that is the interns and residents, are well rested. The new regulations do reduce the chance of physician error, but have instilled in some of them a sense of entitlement to time off, and a feeling of being put-upon if overworked. When they go into practice, they feel (and perhaps they're right) entitled to a liberal on-call schedule in a group practice. The tradeoff is that many of them will have missed their opportunity to participate in some of the essentials of surgical training. There may be gaps, procedures or rare complications they never get to see during their six years of residency, procedures and situations they'll encounter when they start private practice and will be ill-equipped to handle. Somehow though, when they finish their six years of surgical residency they're ready, their brains packed with more medical information than we had access to twenty-five years ago. We just like to complain; it takes the edge off. My cell phone went off. It was Toni on the diabetic floor.

Dr. English was there seeing Annie. I swallowed my tea and went up. English was wrapped in a yellow paper gown, surgical mask, cap, and gloves. Mr. Walker wore a yellow gown as well. Annie's open wound, infected with methacillin-resistant Staph, had made her an isolation patient. No one was allowed in unless he was dressed like a toxic waste disposal worker.

I looked at Annie. Again her eyes welled up. Dr. English had been even more emphatic than I. Mr. Walker became her voice. "How much do you have to take off?"

I had to be frank. "I'll start below the knee, but if there's infection at that level or if the blood supply appears too weak for healing, then I'll have to move up — above the knee." Annie, out of options, took the consent form and signed it without reading it. It occurred to me then that during Annie's entire ordeal, the root of her problem was never mentioned — the type 2 diabetes.

Back at the nurse's station, I phoned Sue at the O.R. desk. She said she'd have an open room in 45 minutes. I checked Annie's preoperative blood work, repeated the blood sugar, 128 mg percent, and paged the intern and the resident to assist me in the O.R. I went back to Annie's room to calm her down, to assure her that she'd be asleep for the entire procedure. I told Mr. Walker I'd see him in the surgical waiting area as soon as I finished. I went to the O.R. locker room and changed into scrubs. As I passed the O.R. desk, Sue informed me that both the intern and resident were tied up with other cases. The only other Sunday surgical resident, the second-year, was tied up too; he was covering the E.R. My assistant would be Henry, a third-year medical student. It's tough to get help on weekends.

Chimera: An Imaginary Monster Composed of Incongruous Parts

I paged Henry to meet me in the doctors' O.R. lounge. He was eager to see an amputation. This would be his first. I grabbed a piece of chalk, erased the graffiti on the blackboard, and prepared to give an impromptu lecture on amputations. I sat down, pondering the hundreds of amputations I'd done over the years. The first operation I ever did, "skin-to-skin," as a supervised surgical resident, was a below-the-knee amputation. As I waited for Henry, my thoughts wandered back to the unnerving experience I'd had the week before. I was leaving a vascular surgical symposium in New York City. It was 5 P.M. The glass-and-steel skyscrapers on 60th Street and Sixth Avenue were disgorging throngs of blue-suited, briefcase-carrying men and smartly dressed women. They carried their coats on that balmy, misplaced afternoon in late October. The women's heels clicked on the mica-flecked sidewalk. Most were heading downtown, their eyes fixed straight ahead. No eye contact in this city.

I was walking uptown. My car was parked on 63rd. At the corner, I stopped to wait for the light. The rush-hour, cross-town traffic whizzed west, providing only momentary glimpses of the crowd waiting to continue downtown. In that crowd, through the fleeting gaps in the traffic, my eye was drawn to a solitary figure. He was in his own space, illuminated by a shaft of setting sunlight. The stoplight turned, the torrent of traffic stopped, but I remained on the curb, transfixed, as the object of my distraction came into focus. At first he looked like a bear: long, bushy, brown hair, wild frizzy beard, and a dirty brown coat. Of course, a homeless man. Not unusual. They say there are twenty thousand in New York City. This one was different though, way different. It was his feet. A battered boot covered the left, but his right foot was orange — neon-orange. It appeared to be the naked, webbed foot of a duck.

I've seen lots of feet. Feet are my business. Vascular surgeons deal with feet all the time. The healthy ones are pink, the bloodless ones are white, and the dead ones are black — but orange? I waited as he lurched toward me, working the skeleton of an umbrella as a cane. He climbed the curb and stopped just in front of me for breath. My eyes traveled down his pant leg to the orange foot. Yes, there was a joint, a right-angle joint, then the flayed-out, short, webbed foot of a duck. I lifted my head. Not polite to stare. He was looking straight at me, face to face. He grinned. "Like it?" he asked. Then he hooked the umbrella over his wrist, pinched each side of his pant leg and, like a teenager flaunting new shoes, pulled up his cuff. Now it was clear — he'd made a prosthesis out of a traffic cone. Ingenious.

Despite his appearance, when he smiled, his eyes twinkled. He seemed friendly, not crazy, no threat in any case. At ankle level the remains of an iridescent ring of reflector tape glowed in the sun. The tip of the orange cone was slit at the back, bent forward, and flayed from wear, which made it webbed. The rush-hour crowd streamed by us; no one turned a head. He looked down, then up, then uttered, "Time for a new one, I guess."

Having removed so many, I know a thing or two about legs and leg prostheses. When all is said and done, a state-of-the-art leg prosthesis, at least here in the U.S., costs between six and ten thousand dollars. "They're free." he said. "Just gotta find the right size; I take a narrow."

"Doesn't it rub on your stump?" I asked.

He jerked his head up. "You a doctor?" he responded.

I nodded as I reached into my pocket. His eyes opened a little wider.

"When did they remove it?" I asked.

"'Bout two years ago, I guess."

Then he pulled the cuff further up. He'd cut off the flat black flange, the part of that sits on the ground. "Socks," he said. "Four layers of socks. And there's no pressure on the end of my stump, the pressure's on the sides, jus like it's supposed to be."

"Are you diabetic?" I asked, instinctively wanting to secure a diagnosis. My question changed the atmosphere, darkened his mood. I was prying.

"Yeah," he spat. "But I can see and I can pee — sugar ain't got the best of me." Then he pressed his umbrella to the pavement, spun on his good foot and started forward. I took the bill from my pocket and handed it to him. He grinned again, then floated off in the rush-hour crowd.

I can't say it out loud — for a physician it's heresy — but this country is in desperate need of universal healthcare.

Henry knew Annie from her previous admission, but hadn't seen her since she'd returned to the E.R. He asked if we were removing her toe. I asked, considering her circulatory status and the condition of her foot, if he thought that a toe amputation would heal. I held the hard copy of the MRA to the window, and pointed to the blocked blood vessels in her calf and lower leg. "I guess not," he said.

I said, "Let's go over the various types of amputations."

The Amputation

In many parts of the world, exploding landmines and improvised explosive devices account for most of the leg amputations. Afghanistan, Angola, and Cambodia lead the list in land mine casualties. It is estimated that in Asia, Africa and the Middle East, over 110 million land mines remain buried in the soil. Many have the potential to explode for up to 50 years. In Africa alone, 37 million land mines are planted like tulip bulbs across 19 countries.[7] Here in the United States, diabetes is the leading cause for any type of amputation — over 80,000 are done each year![8] Studies have shown that diabetics with foot ulcers and poor glucose control — high HbA1c levels — are more likely to undergo amputation than are patients who keep their HbA1c levels in normal range.[9]

I listed the various types of lower-extremity amputation. There are six of them. The level of amputation for a particular patient hinges on two factors: the blood supply, and the level of infection. The goal with most amputations is to save as much of the leg as possible. The surgeon aims for a stump that heals well and fits comfortably into a prosthetic device. We never amputate between bones, through a joint, that is. All joints are lined with cartilage, a tissue with very poor blood suppply. The pressure from walking on the cartilaginous end of a bone results in skin breakdown and poor healing.

I drew the six types of amputations involving the lower extremity on the board:

(1) Partial toe, through any of the small bones, the phalanges, of the toe.

(2) Complete toe (Raye) amputation, which involves removing the entire toe plus the metatarsal head (the end of the metatarsal bone which is attached by a ball joint to the toe).

(3) The transmetatarsal amputation, which (TMA) entails removing all the toes, plus the cartilaginous heads of all the metatarsal bones. It amounts to removal of the forefoot. Before we started doing foot-salvaging bypass grafts, this operation was so common that it was called the diabetic operation.

(4) The Syme amputation, removal of the entire foot through the ankle joint, which is no longer done. The Syme stump can't be fitted to a functional prosthesis, and the skin over the cartilaginous ends of the fibula and tibia is exposed to excessive trauma.

(5) Below the knee, the most common diabetic amputation (BKA). The leg is removed at the mid or lower third of the calf. The BKA stump, if fashioned properly, fits well into an articulated prosthesis. Most people with a BKA prosthesis walk without a limp.

(6) Above the knee amputations (AKA), which are performed on patients who have infection extending into the calf, or above the knee, or have blood supply that's insufficient to heal a BKA (fig. 8).

There is one exception to the rule "save as much as you can." Bedridden patients who have no hope of ever walking are best off with an above the knee amputation even when a below the knee amputation can be expected to heal. Bedridden patients, you see, always fold up their knees; the leg becomes fixed in that folded position, permanently contracted. The stump invariably rubs on the bed sheets, ulcerates, and becomes infected. Eventually they require conversion to an AKA. It's better to do the AKA from the start. One operation is better than two.

Young people who are in reasonably good physical shape can walk with an above the knee prosthesis. Many maneuver quite well, but a lot more energy is required to walk with an AKA prosthesis than with a below the knee prosthesis. So for the weak or elderly, an above the knee amputation often means a wheelchair-bound life.

"So from these X-rays," Henry said, "it looks like Mrs. Walker will need an above the knee amputation."

"It looks that way," I said, "but sometimes the MRA can fool you. I plan to start below the knee, make my incision through the skin and muscle and then assess the bleeding. If the bleeding is brisk and appears adequate to support healing, then I'll continue and Mrs. Walker will end up with a below the knee amputation."

"What if the bleeding is poor?"

"Then I'll have to move up above the knee to the mid-thigh area and do the amputation at that level."

"What if she had gone through the arterial bypass procedure that you first recommended?" he asked.

"Then she would

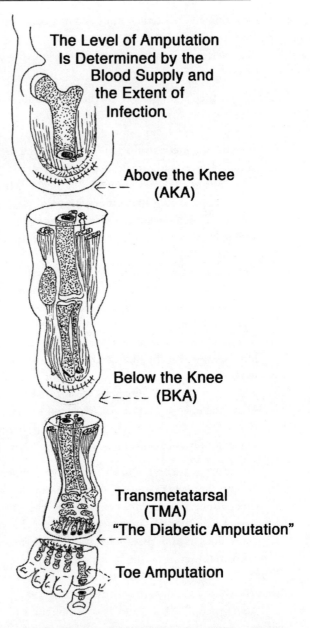

The Level of Amputation Is Determined by the Blood Supply and the Extent of Infection.

Above the Knee (AKA)

Below the Knee (BKA)

Transmetatarsal (TMA) "The Diabetic Amputation"

Toe Amputation

Fig. #8b: Types of amputation in diabetics. In the United States, diabetes accounts for the majority of amputations. The level of amputation depends upon the extent of infection and the blood supply.

likely be home now, with a healing foot ulcer or at worst, an amputated toe."

The phone rang. It was Sue. Annie was there, checked in, and ready to go into room 16.

When we arrived, Dr. Leary, the anesthesiologist, was paging through Annie's chart and asking the usual questions. He raised the possibility of doing a spinal. I reminded him that Annie had positive blood cultures and the possibility of seeding the spinal cord with infected blood from the needle stick should be avoided. By then, I knew Annie well; she needed to be asleep.

Some anesthesiologists ask the patient what type of anesthetic they would like, when instead they should tell the patient what type of anesthetic they need. We wheeled Annie's gurney down the hall into room 16 and positioned it alongside the operating table. Jenny patted the white sheet and beckoned her over. Jenny was just back from maternity leave, but she still looked pregnant. "How's the baby?" I asked.

"Oh, fine, healthy. He weighed in at 8 lbs. 10 oz."

"That's great," I said. I didn't mention that high birth weight babies have a much greater chance of developing type 2 diabetes later in life. I wondered if she'd had gestational diabetes. It occurs in 8 percent of pregnancies, usually in the early part of the third trimester. If she did have gestational diabetes, she'd have better than a 50–50 chance of developing type 2 diabetes later in life.

Jenny's the "gopher," the circulating nurse. She gathers supplies, adjusts the light, mops brows and answers the phone. She gave Annie a pillow and wrapped her with a warm blanket. Dr. Leary took her vital signs and hooked up her EKG leads. I reintroduced her to the masked medical student. She seemed calm, but she wasn't; her heart monitor showed a rate of 125 beats per minute. Leary leaned over Annie's head and whispered, "You'll be fine Annie; we'll take good care of you."

He picked up the IV line, injected Propophill to put her to sleep, then a muscle relaxant to eliminate her gag reflex and ease the placement of his endotracheal tube. He waited about 30 seconds, tilted her head back, opened her mouth with the thumb and index finger of his left hand, inserted his laryngoscope, and gently slid the endotracheal tube between her vocal cords. She didn't move. He squeezed some ointment into each eye, and taped them shut. Jenny placed a foam pad under her good foot. That heel would be resting on the hard table for a while, and the padding would prevent a pressure sore.

Henry and I went out to the scrub sink. We watched through the glass as Jenny soaped Annie's leg from the bandaged foot up to the groin. The scrub nurse, Annette, gave each of us a sterile gown. Jenny tied it in the back; Annette helped us on with our gloves. Jenny lifted the foot by the heel; we painted Annie's leg with brown, Betadine antiseptic, rewrapped the foot with sterile gauze, and finished draping. We were ready to start the amputation. I used a sterile marking pen to outline my "fish-mouth" incision at the mid-calf. Annette handed me the scalpel. I made an incision through the blue ink. It bled! It bled pretty well! I deepened the incision through the subcutaneous tissue, then, using a fresh scalpel, cut through the fascia and into the muscle of the calf, the gastrocnemius.

The bleeding wasn't brisk; no pumping vessels, but it appeared sufficient to allow healing. The muscle was pink, not that grayish pallor you see with blood-starved muscle. "We can stay below the knee," I told Henry. He didn't answer; he was pale and sweating. The edge of his blue paper cap was wet. His glasses were foggy. Jennie rolled a stool behind him. He needed to sit.

"I'm all right," he said. "It's just hot in here."

It wasn't hot. It was cold. "Sit for a minute," I said. "We can wait." I held the dripping wound firmly with two laparotomy pads while we waited for his lightheadedness to pass.

He took a few deep breaths, stood up and said, "I'm okay. It's just hot." Jenny left the stool, just in case.

I continued my dissection, creating long anterior and posterior skin flaps, so that when I closed the incision there would be no tension on the stitches. A small artery began to squirt, a little pink geyser, a good sign. Annette offered me the cautery, a small pen-like electric instrument with a metal tip. A quick buzz and the bleeding would stop. I gave it back. Henry was puzzled. "Why no cautery?" he asked.

"I don't use cautery on diabetics' legs," I replied. "Why add a burn to a wound with shaky blood supply?"

I explained that the cautery cuts and stops bleeding with thermal energy, and even though the burns are minimal, they're still burns, and the diabetic's cauterized tissue doesn't heal as readily as tissue cut with the scalpel. I tied off the bleeding vessel with a fine absorbable ligature. I continued the dissection into the anterior tibial muscles, and the remainder of the gastrocnemius. I encountered the three major arteries: the anterior tibial, the posterior tibial, and the peroneal. I held out my hand; Annette slapped me a clamp. Time to quiz Henry. Could he identify the three arteries? As a third-year student, he should know the anatomy. He got one out of three, the anterior tibial. I held it with my forceps as I dissected it away from the vein, then I asked Henry to pinch it. It was hard, a little lead pipe, so calcified I had to cut it with a heavy scissors. You could hear the crunch. It didn't bleed. It was blocked by plaque. The posterior tibial, solidly calcified too, didn't bleed either. Only the peroneal had a trickle of blood flowing through it. I ligated it with fine absorbable suture.

Almost the entire blood supply to Annie's lower leg arrived through collateral vessels, small unnamed arteries that had enlarged to compensate for the blockage of her three main arteries the blockage caused by her diabetes and her cigarettes. The pencil-sized posterior tibial nerve is the largest nerve in the lower leg. I pulled it down gently with a clamp, then cut it and watched the ends retract like a rubber bands. I cut the fibrous membrane between the tibia and fibula. Then, using my scalpel like a pencil, I drew the blade around each bone, severing the pink periosteum, the sensitive membrane that wraps all bones. The periosteum is the tissue that smarts when you bang your shin. Using a dry gauze sponge, I pushed the cut sheath of periosteum up like a sleeve towards the knee. This exposed the clean white bone.

Now, the two bones alone held the leg in place. I explained to Henry that the fibula must be cut at least an inch higher than the tibia. Otherwise, it will rub against the prosthesis and cause skin ulceration. I showed him how to hold the ankle securely, like a baseball bat, as I sawed through the fibula with the toothed blade of a small reciprocating device. I switched saw blades and severed the tibia, leaving a generous anterior bevel. "You need that bevel," I told him, "so the skin lies smoothly on top of the bone."

Henry was left holding the detached leg. "You can give it to Jennie," I said. Sweat was beading on his forehead. The room was cool. "Are you all right?" I asked.

"Yep, just hot."

Henry used the suction as I irrigated the open stump with sterile saline. Then, using a rasp, I filed smooth the sharp edges of the cut bones. Blood dripped from the marrow cavity of the tibia. I held my thumb against the soft, warm marrow, and pressed. The bleeding stopped. Latex has a hemostatic effect. We were almost ready to close. Annette asked what suture I wanted. "4 / O vicral for the fascia, and 4 / O nylon for the skin," I told her.

I tied off four small pumping vessels, and then held pressure with a dry laparotomy pad until all the bleeding stopped. Then, using the vicral suture, I closed the fascia, the tough fibrous blanket that covers the muscles. This created a protective pad over the bone. Then, without using forceps (they bruise the skin), I gently sutured the stump closed. This created a smile.

I covered the smile with Vaseline gauze, then fluffy gauze pads, and wrapped the stump with a gauze roll. Finally, I bound it firmly with an Ace bandage and placed a Velcro-strapped knee immobilizer around what was left of her leg. The knee immobilizer, I told Henry, would prevent her from flexing her knee joint, a natural reaction to postoperative pain. That can result in a contracture, a folded joint, which is difficult, even with physical therapy, to straighten out. We would keep it on for a few days and then she would start physical therapy.

Annie began to gag from the irritation of the endotracheal tube; the muscle relaxant had worn off. She was waking up. Dr. Leary checked the blood oxygen monitor, satisfied with the reading; he deflated the balloon cuff on the endotracheal tube and pulled it out. He held Annie's head while the four of us moved her to the gurney. We wheeled her, more asleep than awake, to the recovery room. Dr. Leary gave the anesthesia report to Annie's recovery room nurse. Henry and I wrote post-op orders. I requested a stat blood sugar. I noticed that Leary had stopped the insulin drip. It was too much trouble to start another IV line. The blood sugar was 146 mg percent. We restarted the insulin drip. I called her diabetologist. He would control the blood sugars postop.

I left Henry with Annie and went to the waiting room to see Mr. Walker. He was standing at the door, Cousin Linda behind him. "Your wife is fine," I told him, "and we were able to stay below the knee." He forced a smile and nodded.

I explained that that was the best news, since now she should have no trouble walking with a below-the-knee prosthesis. "Encourage her to move in the bed, and take deep breaths from time to time," I said. "It'll help prevent respiratory problems and phlebitis ... and, oh, don't be alarmed if she gets confused again, especially at night. It happens in post-op patients. It's called 'sun-downing.' It's temporary. We'll get a sitter to watch her, if we need to."

Mr. Walker thanked me. Cousin Linda just stood there, silently. I went to the locker room, changed my clothes and headed to the cafeteria for lunch. They had fried chicken legs. I had a salad.

Type 2 Diabetes, a Diagnosis in Need of Respect

After lunch, looking forward to having the rest of Sunday off, I went to my locker to change out of scrubs. Before I could get my locker open, my cell phone rang. This time it was the admissions office, a text message — Would I please come down and sign a death certificate?

"*Whose?*" I wondered. Did one of my patients die while I was in the O.R. with Annie? They all looked good on rounds. My answering service knew I was in the operating room; I'd called them. I picked up the locker room phone and called Admissions. They put me on hold. I waited, and then ... click. I was cut off. I dressed and went down to the little room in the Admissions suite where the death certificates are kept, a trip I've made too many times over the years. The door was closed. I knocked. A woman's voice beckoned me in.

Grace, as usual, was sitting at her desk, thumbing through some papers. "Did you call me?" I asked.

"Yes doctor, you need to fill out this death certificate."

At the risk of sounding callous or uninformed or both, I asked, "Whose death certificate?" She pushed an emergency room chart over the desk. The name on the tab read: "Stephen Krantz."

Steve was a longtime patient of mine. I'd seen him in the office only a few days before. He'd developed a new foot ulcer. He was just 49, an insulin-dependent, type 2 diabetic. He was on dialysis, too, but despite all his problems, he was upbeat and joking. I'd operated on him at least five times in recent years, nothing major — toe amputations, dialysis access problems, a hernia. Gail and I knew that he was noncompliant. He didn't take care of himself. His wife, June, tried to keep him in line, but got nowhere; she couldn't mention his smoking. He was still overweight and although he was on once daily insulin, he rarely checked his blood sugar.

I opened the E.R. chart. He'd been brought in at 5 A.M. with chest tightness, sweating, and low blood pressure. A stat EKG showed a large, new inferior wall myocardial infarction, a big one. The E.R. staff and cardiology fellow were rushing to get him to the cardiac cath lab when he went into sudden cardiac arrest. According to the E.R. doc's note, they worked on him for 45 minutes, but couldn't revive him. His usual cardiologist was off, and they were unable to get hold of his internist, so June suggested they call me for the death certificate. I remembered he had a teenage son and daughter. They were a fairly religious Jewish family, and that accounted for the rush to complete the death certificate. The funeral would be tomorrow.

As I finished reading the chart, I noticed the last sentence of the final note: "Cause of death — acute myocardial infarction." Typical. That's what most doctors would write on the death certificate. Under the "contributing conditions" section were listed hypertension and kidney failure, and chronic dialysis. I knew the real story, though — the average noncompliant, insulin-dependent type 2 diabetic cuts his life short by about twenty years. Subtract eight more years for the average smoker (CDC statistics), add the "nice guy" factor and there we are — dead at 49.

According to research recorded in the February 2006 issue of the journal *Diabetes Care*, diabetes is grossly underestimated as a cause of death. Those who die with a known history of diabetes have the disease listed on their death certificates less than 40 percent of the time.[10] The resulting underestimation of the prevalence of diabetes is important because the National Center for Health Statistics records such data and reports it to the Centers for Disease Control, National Institutes of Health, and other government organizations. These institutions then determine the financial burden of various diseases in the United States. Those statistics are used to promote funding to stimulate public interest and research in the various disease categories. In addition to these skewed statistics, one-third of the world's diabetics are unaware that they even have the disease. So, as they go merrily along untreated, their bodies are undergoing the slow, subtle changes that bring about heart attacks, strokes, kidney failure, and all the other diabetes- induced complications.

Perhaps the national trend towards closure of hospital-based diabetes clinics could be reversed if the true statistics were revealed. Our hospital, the fifth largest in the United States, like many other hospitals, has disbanded its diabetes clinic. It was too costly to run, and the hospital makes a lot more money treating diabetic complications than it can training and paying educators to prevent them.

I filled out the death certificate and jotted down June's home phone number. I would wait a day or two, and then give her a call.

Chapter 7

HEART DISEASE: THE CASE OF GLORIA NUTTER

Gloria Nutter was not conscious when I met her; in fact, her heart wasn't even beating. She was on the operating table, in room number 9. The cardiac surgeons had just completed a four vessel, coronary artery bypass. They were about to take her off the pump; that is, restart her heart with a small electric shock and disconnect her from the cardiopulmonary bypass machine.

It was at that very moment they discovered that her right leg was cold and pulseless. Even her dark skin could not hide the purple mottling which extended from her mid-thigh down to her toes. They felt her right groin. No pulse there either. They felt her left leg; it was warm with a loud Doppler pulse in the foot. They concluded that while they were fixing her heart, her right iliac artery, just above the groin, had become obstructed. The blockage was probably a clot, or perhaps a piece of plaque had broken off from where they were working and had lodged, like a log in a brook, in a narrow part in the vessel. They needed a peripheral vascular surgeon right away.

A surgeon's day is never routine. One emergency can turn a well-planned day into a marathon; and if it comes before office hours, a frazzled nurse must push twenty-five peeved patients to another day. It happens a lot. It happened the day the cardiac surgeon called me in to fix Gloria's leg. It was a neatly planned day, three surgeries in the morning, lunch if there was time, and 2 P.M. office hours. I'd finished the first case, a gall bladder, and was between a breast and a hemorrhoid when the call came in.

The cardiac surgeons gave me a quick history: Gloria was a type 2 diabetic on insulin, who eight years previously had suffered a stroke when atherosclerotic plaque filled her left carotid artery. The stroke left her with paralysis of the right arm and leg, and with an inability to speak. After months of physical therapy, the leg and arm function returned, but despite intensive speech therapy she remained, for the most part, mute. She had aphasia. The stroke had permanently damaged the part of her brain that controls the ability to talk. That didn't keep her from trying though, for she knew exactly what she wanted to say; the words just wouldn't come out.

I observed, days after her surgery, that she could say "yes" and "no." However, when she wanted to say "yes," "no" came out; and when she wanted to say "no," "yes" came out. When she attempted to speak, her face would flush, her eyes would tear, and her mouth would open like a fish's gasping for air. Occasionally, a word or two would escape, but then, frustrated, she would close her mouth, drop her shoulders and stop trying.

The cardiac surgeons restarted her heart without difficulty, and then they took her off cardiac bypass. Her systolic blood pressure rose from 90 mm of mercury, normal for a patient on a cardiopulmonary bypass pump, to 140 mm of mercury and remained stable. Her right leg, however, remained pulseless and cold.

Taking her history into account, and knowing she'd already been on the operating room table for over four hours, I decided that she was not a candidate for an extensive intra-abdominal operative procedure. There are other, less invasive ways to remedy a blocked iliac artery. I would reestablish blood flow to her right leg by the simplest means possible; I'd remove the clot from below, through a right groin incision. I would expose the pulseless femoral artery, open it, and pass a balloon-tipped catheter through and above the clot, then inflate the balloon and pull the catheter out, extracting the clot with the dime-sized balloon tip.

If that didn't work, if the balloon-tipped catheter could not be passed through the obstructed artery, then I would do a simple bypass using a synthetic Dacron tube, 6 mm in diameter (about the width of a cigarette), to shunt the blood from the left femoral artery into my opening in the right femoral artery below the obstruction. The Dacron graft would be tunneled under the skin, in a slight arc just above the pubic bone, from the left femoral artery to the right. This would detour the blood supply around the obstruction and avoid the need for an amputation. I asked the circulating nurse to page my surgical resident. I needed assistance. He was busy. He sent Frank, the intern.

While one cardiac surgeon began closing the chest, his partner went off to the cardiac waiting area to find Mrs. Nutter's family. He would explain to them that the cardiac procedure went well, but during the operation a problem had arisen. The blood supply to right leg had become blocked, and we would be another hour or two fixing it.

I attempted to extract the clot from below, using the balloon-tipped catheter, but I couldn't get the catheter through the obstruction. This was more than a simple, soft clot. I resorted to doing the left femoral to right femoral artery bypass graft. It took a while, but it went without a hitch. When the Dacron graft was sewn in place and the two arteries were connected, I removed the vascular clamps. With the replenished blood supply, within a few seconds the leg warmed up, the skin mottling disappeared, and Doppler pulses returned to the foot.

There was some minor bleeding at the graft-to-artery suture line, the anastomosis; a few extra sutures stopped it. We closed the two incisions layer by layer, placed a dressing, and wheeled Gloria, still intubated, to the recovery room. I asked the recovery room nurses to do a quick finger stick blood sugar. It was 260. Unfortunately, many anesthesiologists — who rarely see their patients again once they leave the operating room — are unaware of the benefits gained with continuous insulin drips to control intraoperative blood sugar. So many anesthesiologists never learn that continuous IV insulin drips during surgery can better control blood sugar levels, and this results in fewer postoperative complications like wound infections, and respiratory, kidney and neurological problems. I ordered the insulin drip and explained my part of the procedure to the recovery room nurses. Then I went to the cardiac surgery waiting area to meet Gloria's family.

Gloria's son and daughter were sitting in the corner, eyes focused on the door. It had been more than six hours since they had seen their mother wheeled into the operating room. The receptionist pointed them out. I went over, pulled up a chair, and we talked. They explained that they had been caring for Gloria for eight years, since the stroke. Barbara, the daughter, lived with her, but she worked, so Gloria was alone for most of the day. They followed a strict routine set by their internist for blood sugar testing, diet, and the administration of insulin. Barbara said her mother had no trouble getting around the house. However, when they took her out she managed to walk only to the corner, about half a block. Then she'd have to rest until the pain in her right leg subsided before turning around and walking back.

"What prompted the visit to the cardiac surgeon?" I asked.

"When she went for her usual checkup," Barbara said, "the doctor found ominous changes in her EKG. He sent her for more tests and a cardiac angiogram; two days later, here we are."

"Did she have any heart symptoms? Shortness of breath, chest pain?" I asked.

"No, but she sleeps in a chair, sort of sitting up."

"Does she have trouble breathing when she lies flat?"

"She never lies flat. If she tries to, her right foot aches. That's why she sleeps in a chair — so she can keep her foot on the carpet."

"That explains the problem in the O.R.," I said. "She had rest pain. When she lies flat in bed, she loses the effect of gravity pulling more blood to the feet, so she sits and the pain subsides."

People with rest pain often sleep in a chair or hang their foot over the side of the bed. It's their only way of getting relief. Pain of any type is worse at night. During the day, when the mind is occupied, low level pain is masked by various sensations and external stimuli, and is easier to ignore. At night, when everything is quiet and the body's at rest, even minor pain is amplified to the point of distraction.

So it was clear to me now that the leg problem was, to a large extent, present prior to the heart surgery. When the cardiac surgeons put her on a pump (a cardiopulmonary bypass), her blood pressure, normally about 180/85, fell to 90/60. That alone would make the leg cold and pulseless. Add the effect of lying flat for four hours and the result is a dying extremity.

I reassured Barbara and her brother and went back to the recovery room. Gloria was still asleep, still on the respirator, in an intentionally induced pharmacologic coma. They'd arouse her later in the day when her vital signs stabilized. I checked her feet; the soles were warm and pink.

The following morning I made the cardiac recovery room my first stop. During the night Gloria had been extubated. The breathing tube was removed, and she was taken off the respirator. Her vital signs, blood pressure, pulse and respirations were stable. Her blood sugar was 110. She was on her insulin drip. Her femoral artery graft was open; I could feel it pulsating beneath her skin. She looked good. She was lying comfortably, flat in the bed. I asked, "Do you feel okay?"

She opened her mouth and shook her head "yes," but out came "no." Then, "I... I... I..." She closed her mouth, looked straight at me, and shook her head "yes" again.

I asked if her foot hurt. She smiled and shook her head, "no." I wrote my note in her chart and continued my rounds.

The following day, she was transferred out of the cardiac ICU and into a semi-private room. The other bed, the one by the window, was occupied by an obtundent octogenarian who spoke continually to someone who did not exist. Gloria didn't seem to mind; she smiled and answered my questions with a nod.

By the fifth day post-op, Gloria was ready to go home. I'd arranged that her nurse page me when the family arrived so I could give them a plan for post-op care and office follow-up. At 10:30 A.M. the ward clerk, Trish, called. I was almost finished placing a skin graft on the leg of a lady with a pancake sized ulceration on the anterior surface of her shin. "Could they wait 20 minutes?" I asked through the O.R. speakerphone.

When I arrived, Barbara, the daughter, was sitting in the recliner and Gloria was shoeless on the bed, but dressed and ready to leave. They were both smiling. Barbara was clutching a bunch of prescriptions left by the cardiac surgeons.

I felt Gloria's feet. They were both warm. The right foot now had palpable pulse at the ankle. I checked her groin incisions, and then I gave Gloria and her mother instructions for post-op care and a date for follow-up in my office. Barbara thanked me, turned to her mother and asked, "Did you want to say something to the doctor, Mama?"

Gloria, now sitting on the side of the bed, looked up, squinted, opened her mouth and out came, "I... I... I'm...I'm... *internally* grateful."

Barbara looked at me and smiled.

Heart disease and the diabetic patient.

There is an old medical adage which was inspired by third-year medical students upon reaching that pivotal moment when they must choose a medical specialty. Surgery? Pediatrics? Internal medicine? The saying goes: "Surgeons do everything, but know nothing. Internists know everything, but do nothing. Psychiatrists know nothing and do nothing. And pathologists do everything and know everything — but one day too late."

This exaggerated aphorism forces us to acknowledge the faults in our profession — that there is a disconnect between medical specialties. The practice of medicine has become so specialized that when your disease requires the input of several different specialists, the continuity of care may become disrupted; there may be lapses in communication that result in superfluous testing and unrecognized patient needs. The end result is expensive medical care and slipshod treatment. The American Diabetes Association stresses that diabetic patients, in view of their multifaceted medical problems, be treated by a coordinated team of physicians and educators rather than by individual practitioners. Better communication and cross-training between specialties is needed, but is unfortunately unavailable under our current healthcare system.

Had the cardiac surgeons who operated on Gloria known enough about the treatment of diabetes, they would have had her on an insulin drip throughout her operation. Gloria benefited from her internist's knowledge of cardiology and from the expertise of her cardiac surgeons. As a result, she was a happy statistic, but for want of a little extra knowledge of a very common disease, she might have become a sad statistic. Her cardiologist was aware that one third of type 2 diabetics with cardiac disease are asymptomatic; they may have no overtly recognizable sign of heart disease, yet they may have significant coronary artery blockages, silent coronary artery disease. The mere presence of Gloria's peripheral vascular disease, her claudication and rest pain, was a good clue that she might have coronary artery disease as well. That she had no symptoms of heart disease was not surprising, because in the type 2 diabetic, typical cardiac symptoms are often erased by neuropathy.[1] But autonomic nerve dysfunction (autonomic neuropathy) affects the hearts of many diabetics and may in itself be a cause for silent cardiac disease. Here, insufficient blood is pumped through the coronary arteries, even when the coronary arteries are not blocked by atherosclerotic plaque. This form of silent coronary artery disease, like that caused by blocked coronary arteries, may be detected by a stress test. Potential heart failure or heart attacks can be prevented with statin drugs, aspirin, lifestyle changes to improve diet, and monitored exercise.

Diabetes-related heart disease may take different forms in different parts of the world. In sub–Saharan Africa, for example, type 2 diabetics are particularly prone to heart disease but, unlike diabetic heart disease in the U.S., the coronary arteries are often not clogged. Africans are genetically prone to *cardiomyopathy*— decreased heart muscle function in the absence of coronary artery disease or hypertension.[2] This condition is associated with cardiac enlargement and progressive symptomatic congestive heart failure. The rising incidence of type 2 diabetes in Africa is, once again, due to the adoption of the American lifestyle and eating habits. And in Africa it's compounded by the lowest doctor/patient ratio in the populated world. Sixty-seven percent of diabetic patients in sub–Saharan Africa die of heart disease.

Many Americans are diagnosed with a combination of conditions which together are called "the metabolic syndrome." This syndrome consists of any three of the following: abdominal obesity, high blood pressure, an elevated triglyceride level, low levels of HDL (good cholesterol), or glucose intolerance. People with this syndrome are at particularly high risk to develop heart attacks, strokes and peripheral vascular occlusive disease. Diabetics with this syndrome have an exceptionally high risk for heart attacks. The risks are reduced with weight loss, exercise (if cleared by the doctor), statins (cholesterol lowering drugs), and blood pressure lowering medications.

Presently, the American Diabetes Association recommends that all type 2 diabetics over the age of forty take statin therapy (anti–LDL, or bad cholesterol, drugs) *regardless* of the presence or absence of cardiovascular disease and even if their base line LDL cholesterol levels are normal.[3] This recommendation seems reasonable since LDL cholesterol is the primary factor in clogging coronary arteries which cause heart attacks, and heart attacks are the major cause of death in the diabetic. There are, however, some studies that argue that this approach may be unwarranted in diabetics whose baseline cholesterol levels are normal, and in those who have no existing coronary artery disease.

Diabetics in the U.S. have four times the heart attack rate of non-diabetics, and when they do have a heart attack, the mortality rate is twice that of non-diabetics.[4] Because of the extremely high incidence of coronary artery disease in diabetics, they become candidates for cardiac surgery or angioplasty in greater numbers than the general population. The immediate success rate for these diabetic patients is good, however long term survival and the need for repeat cardiac procedures is increased in the diabetic population. One reason for this is diabetics' propensity for accelerated atherosclerosis. Another is their tendency to clot abnormally.

In scientific terms, the biochemistry of the clotting process is described as a complex cascade of biochemical events. Forming a clot is basically a response to an injury of a blood vessel wall. If the clotting process, this cascade of chemical reactions, is altered by the absence of any particular biochemical component, say fibrinogen, then a clot does not form and bleeding ensues. If there is an excess of one of the ingredients required for clot formation, platelets for example, then accelerated, or pathological clotting, may take place. Diabetics tend to have an excess of fibrinogen and other clotting factors.

All surgery, no matter how minimally invasive it is, inevitably causes collateral tissue damage. The fragile lining of blood vessels, the endothelium, when cut, crushed with a clamp or dilated too vigorously with a balloon during an angioplasty, initiates a natural series of events, designed by nature to stop bleeding; it clots. A blood vessel severed in two, even a fairly large artery, will bleed initially, but the bleeding will quickly stop, because the two ends will contract as if ligated with a stitch. However, if the vessel is partially cut, the rent will be pulled apart by the muscular arterial wall, and unless the opening is small, the bleeding will not stop on its own.

Here's a trick question for medical students: What are the first two branches of the aorta? Answer: The coronary arteries. It's a trick question because the coronary arteries don't look like branches. They spring out from under two aortic valve cusps and remain embedded on the surface of the heart. But the heart, like every other muscle, gets its blood supply from arteries that branch off the aorta. All heart attacks, myocardial infarctions, are caused by the blockage of a segment of a coronary artery. As a result, the corresponding portion of heart muscle receives inadequate oxygen and dies. Everyone has two major coronary arteries: the left main coronary artery and the right coronary artery. Both have major branches. The left circumflex coronary artery supplies oxygenated blood to the left ventricle, and the right circumflex carries blood to the right ventricle (see fig. 9). Small interconnecting arterial branches serve to shunt blood around narrowed or blocked segments of coronary arteries, thus limiting the size of some heart attacks. The classic "drop-dead heart attack" occurs when the blockage involves the beginning of the left anterior descending artery. This artery supplies oxygenated blood to the pumping left ventricle.

There is a characteristic difference in the pattern of coronary artery blockage in diabetics from the pattern of blockage in nondiabetics. In diabetics, blockages tend to occur in multiple areas and primarily at the ends of the coronary arteries, whereas in nondiabetics there tend to be fewer areas of blockage and they usually occur in the proximal or middle part of the artery (see fig. 10).

In recent years, the introduction of coronary artery stenting has provided a less invasive method than open-heart surgery to widen blocked coronary arteries The stenting procedure is called percutaneous transluminal coronary angioplasty (PTCA); it involves threading a balloon-tipped catheter into the narrow segment of the coronary artery, inflating the balloon in order to dilate the artery, and then placing a metal, spring-like stent in the dilated area to keep the vessel open. It is important to note that the mere presence of a severely blocked coronary artery, even if it causes chest pain (angina) is not necessarily an indication for coronary artery stenting or open-heart surgery. Cardiac specialists are of the opinion that the average coronary artery disease patient, with or without exertional angina, diabetic or not, is apt to do just as well if treated medically

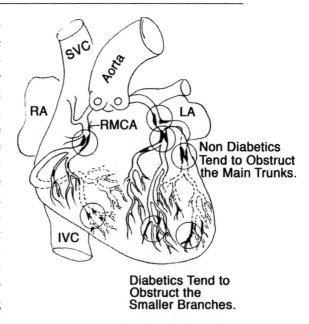

Fig. #9: Coronary artery disease. The leading cause of death in diabetics is heart disease — blocked coronary arteries. Heart attacks are four times more common in diabetics and twice as deadly as in the normal population. Diabetics tend to obstruct the smaller branch arteries, whereas non-diabetics tend to obstruct the main coronary arteries.

with cholesterol-lowering drugs, blood pressure control, clot prevention (aspirin) and monitoring by the cardiologist. You see, heart attacks may not actually occur at the point of maximal narrowing of the coronary artery. Smaller plaques may rupture and result in an acute coronary blockage, and the stenting procedure is not without risk.

According to the American Heart Association, when done during the course of a heart attack, coronary stenting is often a life-saving procedure. Many heart attack victims can attest to that. Timing is everything. If the heart attack victim can be transported to a hospital equipped with a cardiac lab, and receive a stent within an hour of his attack, then he is likely to avoid permanent cardiac muscle damage and longterm disability. Prophylactic stent placement is justified for incapacitating angina or as a precaution prior to major, non-heart related, surgical procedures. In this case,

The Normal Heart

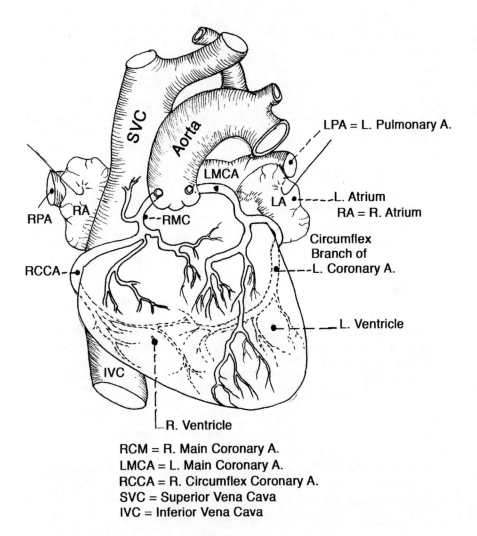

LPA = L. Pulmonary A.

L. Atrium
RA = R. Atrium

Circumflex
Branch of
L. Coronary A.

L. Ventricle

R. Ventricle

RCM = R. Main Coronary A.
LMCA = L. Main Coronary A.
RCCA = R. Circumflex Coronary A.
SVC = Superior Vena Cava
IVC = Inferior Vena Cava

Fig. #10: The anatomy and blood supply of the normal heart.

severe coronary artery blockage presents a risk of heart attack during or
following the surgery. Diabetics have an increased risk of postoperative or
intraoperative heart attacks. This was the reason for preoperative stenting
in Annie Walker's case.

You must remember that there are two types of cardiologists—*inva-*

sive and *noninvasive.* If you are sent to an invasive cardiologist with a significantly blocked coronary artery, then you will likely receive a coronary artery stent in spite of the risks. If you see a noninvasive cardiologist, you are likely to be treated with medications. Ideally, invasive and non-invasive cardiologists should work together to decide what's best for the patient.

Hospitals that offer therapeutic or diagnostic cardiac catheterization procedures should always have a backup cardiac surgery team in the same building, but this is not always the case. Some hospitals have cardiac cath labs, but no cardiac surgeons. It is still legal, and apparently acceptable to the Joint Committee on Hospital Accreditation, for a hospital to run a cardiac catheterization lab without backup cardiac surgical capability. In other words, when a complication occurs during a cardiac catheterization, a cardiac surgeon should be on hand to fix it. For example, if a catheter balloon perforates a coronary artery, resulting in the need for immediate surgical repair, if the hospital has no cardiac surgery service, then that patient must be rushed by ambulance to a properly equipped hospital for emergency surgery. These delays significantly reduce a patient's chances for survival. Choose your hospital carefully.

Many heart attacks are the result of a spontaneous rupture of a coronary artery plaque. This may occur during vigorous activity, or occasionally at rest. Because plaques, lipid and cholesterol filled bumps on the internal surface of the artery, are prone to rupture when the heart is beating rapidly, say when shoveling snow or using the treadmill, people ask, "Why take the risk? Why exercise?" This question has been answered by leading researchers in the field of heart disease. The most famous study, the Framingham Heart Study, concludes that people who are active and include exercise on a routine basis have a longer life expectancy and are more likely to be free of type 2 diabetes.[5] Diabetics who exercise on a routine basis are doubly rewarded because exercise increases insulin sensitivity and lowers baseline sugar levels. The decision to exercise, however, deserves scrutiny. The word "exercise" should always be preceded by the word "sensible," and the sedentary individual, diabetic or not, should be checked by a cardiologist prior to starting an exercise routine.

The stenting procedure, of necessity, injures the tender endothelial lining of the artery. Type 2 diabetics, because of their abnormal clotting tendencies, suffer more complications from this procedure than nondiabetics. The remedy for this potential undesirable clotting is the use of anticoagulants, potent ones at first: Heparin, then Coumadin or aspirin-type drugs for the longterm. The lay term "blood thinner" is often used in place of the proper word "anticoagulant." Anticoagulants, in fact, do not actually alter the viscosity, or "thin" the blood. They simply keep it from clotting by altering the biochemical process of the clotting mechanism. Heparin is a fast acting, injectable anticoagulant. It's used to prevent clotting during open-heart, vascular, and catheter based (stent placement, etc.) surgeries. It is usually administered by injection directly into the bloodstream and produces its anticoagulant effect within minutes, thereby allowing the vascular surgeon to proceed without worrying about clotting. When no longer needed, its effect can be reversed rapidly with a drug called Protamine.

Coumadin, the second type of anticoagulant, is long-acting. It's taken by mouth or initially by injection and requires several days to reach its full effect. Coumadin is primarily used to prevent clotting in people with abnormal heart rhythms, usually atrial fibrillation; as prophylaxis against clotting in patients with artificial heart valves; and for prevention of clot extension in deep vein thrombosis (DVT). The anticoagulant effect of Coumadin can be intentionally reversed with oral or injected vitamin K, which takes up to a few days (or unintentionally by eating too many green leafy vegetables), or with intravenous fresh frozen plasma, which carries a small risk of hepatitis, but stops the anticoagulant effect with in minutes. When a patient on Coumadin requires emergency surgery, say for example an appendectomy or repair of a compound fracture, then fresh frozen plasma is given to reverse the Coumadin effect.

The third commonly used type of anticoagulant works by interfering with platelet function. Platelets are small particles, fragments of bone marrow cells, which find their way into the bloodstream and play a major role in initiating the clotting process. The most common anti-platelet drug, aspirin, has a weak anticoagulant effect. We usually stop aspirin a few days before surgery if possible, but in an emergency the troublesome capillary oozing from impaired platelet function is tolerable for both the. surgeon and the patient. The other major platelet inhibiting-drug, Clopidogrel, is marketed under the name Plavix. I have found it unsafe to operate on people who are taking this drug. Excessive bleeding occurs. The antidote is a transfusion of large quantities of platelets previously obtained from multiple donors and stored frozen in the hospital blood bank. The platelets are defrosted and transfused immediately before and during the operative procedure. Plavix may save lives, but unfortunately there is no good test to measure its effectiveness. Everyone takes the same dose, 75 mgm.[6] This may be too much for some people or too little for others. Moreover, stopping it suddenly may cause a rebound effect that results in excessive clotting and heart attacks — just what it's meant to prevent. The drug must be tapered off.

The three categories of anticoagulants described above do not dissolve clots; they simply prevent clot formation. Thrombolytic agents are another category of drugs. These can be injected directly into the bloodstream to actually dissolve a clot. To be effective, thrombolytics must be used immediately, within minutes, after the clot forms. Thrombolytic agents are useful in treating acute heart attacks and some acute strokes. Their effectiveness is directly related to the time elapsed between the heart attack or stroke and the injection of the drug, or, simply put, how quickly the patient gets to the hospital and how efficient the emergency room is.

Surgeons have an operating room expression, "better is the enemy of good." That is to say, if what you've done looks good and works (for example, a suture repair of a lacerated blood vessel), then don't try to make it look better — you may end up making a bloody mess. Diabetologists have long maintained that blood sugar control, maintaining a HbA1c of 7 percent, is a good way to avoid the longterm complications of diabetes. More specifically, according to research in the United Kingdom, heart attack rates among type 2 diabetics can be reduced by 14 percent for every 1 percent reduction of HbA1c.[7] So why not, they asked, try to achieve even better blood sugar control and thereby reduce the heart attack rate even further? Let's lower the target HbA1c to 6 percent, they thought! That would require intensive, multiple-drug therapy. The researchers rounded up more than 10,000 diabetics with known cardiac disease and, over a period of three and a half years, treated them intensively, striving to get their HbA1c levels below 6 percent. However, when it became obvious that the intensively treated diabetics failed to benefit, and in fact they had a higher death rate than with standard treatment, the researchers stopped the study.[8] Conclusion: In medicine, "better" often is the enemy of "good."

Chapter 8

KIDNEY FAILURE: THE CASE OF BILL MURPHY

Back in the cafeteria on Monday morning at 6:15, I paged my surgical resident. Henry, the med student, answered. He explained that Sanjieve was in the middle of a dressing change, and that all my patients appeared to be stable and, "Oh, yes," he said, "your patient Mrs. Walker, she's confused again."

"Who's scrubbing on my 7:30 case, Mrs. Grasso?" I asked.

"Me. I am," he said.

"Good." I said. "We'll see her first, then Mrs. Walker, then the rest of the patients between cases."

Mrs. Grasso was in the diabetic unit too, in a semi-private room, three doors down from Annie Walker. She and I were old friends. We met years ago in the emergency room. She'd come in with kidney failure and her nephrologist called me to place an emergency hemodialysis catheter. Mrs. Grasso didn't know at the time that she was diabetic. About 20 percent of diabetics learn they have the disease only when they develop a complication from it.

In her case, it wasn't simply the diabetes that caused her kidneys to fail. She had high blood pressure, and a series of urinary tract infections as well. Anyone can get a urinary tract infection, but they occur more often and they're more severe in diabetics. The kidney's function is to filter the blood, to keep the red and white blood cells, protein, and nutrients in, while ridding the body of excess water and nitrogenous waste.

The medical term for kidney disease in diabetics is *diabetic nephropathy*. Over the course of time, diabetes affects the blood vessels more than any other part of the body. I think of the kidneys as two giant clusters of blood vessels. The micro-anatomical complexity of the kidneys, with their many modified vascular structures — the glomeruli, semi-permeable capillary membranes, and specialized tubular cells — make the diabetic's kidneys an easy target. In the United States, chronic progressive kidney failure ranks second to heart disease as the cause of death in diabetics.[1] In undeveloped countries, except parts of Africa, infection is the leading cause of death. Fortunately, diabetics can slow down the progression of kidney failure by carefully controlling their blood pressure with specific medications, tightly restricting the intake of protein, excess fluids, and potassium, and by controlling blood sugar — avoiding dips and elevations. Protein restriction keeps the toxic nitrogenous waste products, measured by the serum blood urea nitrogen level (BUN), to a minimum. Fluid restriction helps avoid heart failure, edema, and high blood pressure. And by keeping the potassium (K) low, diabetics with kidney failure can steer clear of sudden, serious, sometimes fatal, changes in heart rhythm. The electrical conduction system of the heart is extremely sensitive to high blood levels of potassium. A level over 6mEq/cc. can cause sudden death.

Pharmaceutical companies, medical schools, and biomedical research facilities frequently, and often inhumanely, use experimental animals — dogs, monkeys, turtles (they have very sensitive hearts) and other animals — for research or training. Often, at the end of the experiment, the animals are put down, "sacrificed" in the lab. A common method of "sacrifice" is to inject them intravenously with lethal doses of potassium. This stops their hearts instantly, mid-beat. Potassium chloride injected IV is the execution method du jour for those on death row.

Potassium levels rise quickly in diabetics with kidney failure. This puts them at risk for fatal cardiac arrhythmias or cardiac arrest. Excessively high blood potassium levels demand emergency dialysis treatment. In order to administer emergency hemodialysis, the patient requires reliable access to his circulatory system; a catheter must be placed in a large vein. That's how I met Mrs. Grasso; it is my job as the vascular surgeon to insert this pencil-sized catheter into either the internal jugular vein in the neck, or the femoral vein in the groin. The catheter functions as a blood vessel that connects the patient to an artificial kidney, the dialysis machine.

That emergency room visit was years ago, but I still remember her discomfort, her nausea, her vomiting and her complaining of a sudden weight gain. She was visibly short of breath and she said her skin itched terribly. Her laboratory findings confirmed both the diabetes and the kidney failure. Her blood sugar was about 490, and her urinalysis showed 4 plus sugar. She had a BUN of 90. Normal is less than 23. The BUN is a measure of the nitrogenous waste that her kidneys are unable to remove. The weight gain was from retained water. Her potassium was 6.8 mEq per cc.; normal in our lab is less than 4.5.

Simple blood tests, repeated regularly, can determine how well your kidneys are working. The most accurate measure of kidney function, more accurate than the BUN, is the serum creatinine level. Hers was 8 mg percent; normal is below 4.5 mg percent. She was in kidney failure and her K (potassium) was dangerously elevated. Her high serum potassium level alarmed the nephrologist. She needed immediate hemodialysis. That was 10 years, and for her, three operations ago.

If Mrs. Grasso's kidney failure had been caught earlier, she could have avoided that catheter in her jugular vein, that emergency dialysis. I placed that temporary jugular catheter right there in the emergency room, using local anesthesia. The dialysis treatment she received that night dropped her potassium to a safe 4.9 mEq per cc. Her breathing eased after two pounds of excess fluid were intentionally removed during the treatment, and her BUN dropped to 40. The nausea stopped. It was a temporary fix. The next day, in order to prepare her for ongoing dialysis treatments — kidney failure in the diabetic is permanent — she braved a second series of operations, the creation of an arteriovenous, or AV fistula in her left wrist, placement of a Permcath dialysis catheter in her left jugular vein and removal of the temporary dialysis catheter that I had placed the night before. Mrs. Grasso had end-stage kidney failure and now her life would hinge on three dialysis treatments a week (see fig. 13).

Mrs. Grasso is one of a half million people in the United States who, in order to stay alive, must have dialysis three times a week, year after year. Each treatment should last at least four hours. For the first two months, the dialysis nurse attached her to the dialysis machine using the Permcath, the one we planted in her left jugular vein. After that, her treatments were administered through the arteriovenous fistula that we created in her left arm. The preferred type of vascular access, the longest lasting and least prone to infection or clotting problems, is the arteriovenous fistula (AV). An AV fistula is a surgically created connection between a small artery and an adjacent vein (fig. 13). This connection, just under the skin, and only six or seven mm long, allows arterial blood to flow directly into an adjacent vein, bypassing the capillary bed. The high pressure flow from the artery dilates the vein and makes it vibrate like a little motor under the skin. We call the palpable vibration a "thrill." The thrill helps the dialysis nurse find and puncture the enlarged vein six times a week, twice for each dialysis treatment. One needle is inserted to draw the blood out and the other returns it to the patient after it passes through the machine.

As soon as Mrs. Grasso's fistula was ready to use, I removed her Permcath. Without it, she could shower again. But, most importantly, the constant threat of a bloodstream infection was eliminated. That catheter protruding from her neck was no different than a giant splinter.

About 40 percent of diabetics have some degree of kidney damage. They may have no symptoms early on, so all diabetics must have their kidney function followed closely by their internist, endocrinologist, or nephrologist. A urinalysis may show the presence of protein in the urine and blood tests will show a slow rise in the BUN (blood urea nitrogen) and an elevation of the creatinine levels. A third test,

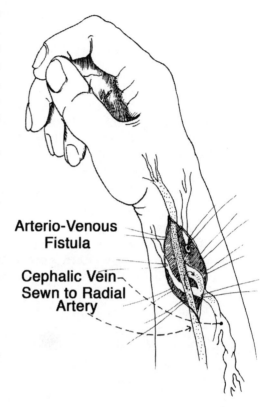

Arterio-Venous Fistula

Cephalic Vein Sewn to Radial Artery

Fig. #13: Arterio-venous fistula. There are several methods to prepare a patient for permanent, tri-weekly hemodialysis. The most reliable, longest-lasting, and least prone to infection and clotting is the AV fistula. There are several variations, but the one most preferred is done in the non-dominant wrist by sewing the radial artery to the cephalic vein. This results in high pressure flow which dilates the vein and allows it to be punctured twice for each dialysis treatment.

the creatinine clearance, may be done to more clearly define the extent of kidney damage. Fortunately, kidney damage progresses slowly in the diabetic, but the decline may go unnoticed until it reaches "end-stage" and the kidneys can no longer sustain life. Then dialysis becomes mandatory.

Kidney damage in the diabetic is not reversible, but it is controllable for a long while. The damage can be held in check by adjusting the diet, controlling blood pressure with appropriate medications, and investigating any signs of urinary tract infection. Periodic renal function tests are vital. And it is most important to avoid dips and elevations in the blood sugar through dietary control, exercise and proper use of oral medications or insulin.

Had Mrs. Grasso known she was a diabetic, she'd have been seeing a doctor who would have referred her to a nephrologist, a kidney specialist. When her blood tests, her creatinine or potassium levels reached a certain point, the kidney specialist would have anticipated the impending need for dialysis. He would have referred her to the vascular surgeon and the AV fistula would have been placed months before she actually required that first dialysis treatment. She could have avoided that emergency room visit 10 years before. She could have avoided the discomfort of having those temporary dialysis catheters placed in her jugular veins. When the time came, when dialysis treatments became mandatory, she would have been prepared.

I found Mrs. Grasso sitting in the chair by her bed. She was staring at her arm. I hadn't seen her for many years; had we met on the street I wouldn't have recognized her. She explained that following her last dialysis, while the nurse was holding pressure to stop the bleeding from the puncture sites, her fistula had clotted; the thrill disappeared. She wasn't happy. "That nurse," she said. "She always presses too hard. I knew one of these times it would clot."

I looked at her arm. There were multiple healing puncture wounds, purple blotches (eccymoses), and the large, tortuous, pulseless veins of a clotted fistula. It looked like a snake had crawled under her skin and died. "You're lucky," I said. "Your dialysis access lasted 10 years. Most people aren't that fortunate."

"I guess so," she said.

She was an experienced dialysis patient. She'd seen many patients in the dialysis unit undergo multiple procedures, usually emergency catheter placements. Bloodstream infections, usually Staphylococcal, are common in patients with protruding dialysis catheters. Sometimes patients in her dialysis shift for years would disappear and never return.

"What are you going to do?" she asked. "I can't miss my next treatment."

I held out her well-used arm. "See this vein up here, the one next to your biceps muscle? That's your cephalic vein. It's near empty now, but it's nice and big from the arterial blood flowing through it all these years. Fortunately, they've never punctured it. I'm going to disconnect it here at the elbow and use it to make a new fistula. I'll plug it into your brachial artery, right here, above the elbow crease. They should be able to use it tomorrow, as long as they stay away from my suture line."

"You mean I won't need a temporary catheter?"

"No, I think we can avoid that."

I checked her chart. Her blood chemistries were normal except for the creatinine of 7.1 and the BUN of 43. It was the potassium (K) I was looking for. It was 5.1 mEq/L — below the danger level. She could hold out one day without dialysis with no ill effect. I called her nephrologist and told him that I'd get her on the O.R. schedule that evening, following office hours. He agreed.

I returned to Mrs. Grasso's room with a surgical consent form, turned it over, and drew a little diagram of the intended procedure on the back. She looked it over and signed it. Toni, her nurse, watched and counter-signed. It's the law; all consent forms must be witnessed. I wrote orders for a low-protein, low-potassium, liquid breakfast, and put her on an insulin drip. I explained that I would operate under local anesthesia and the anesthesiologist would give her some sedation. She was happy with that.

"Will you call the outpatient dialysis unit, or do I call?" she asked.

"They've already been informed. They know you were admitted, but I'll call and let them know you'll be back on Thursday."

"Please, will you ask them to let Bill know I'll be back Thursday, usual shift?"

"Sure," I said.

Annie Walker's Postop Course

After seeing Mrs. Grasso, I walked three doors down to see Annie Walker. It was her first post-operative day. Mr. Walker hadn't arrived yet; it was early. The sitter, one of the nursing aides who usually worked days, had been with her all night. The aide was sitting in the chair next to the bed. She rubbed her eyes and said, "Mrs. Walker's been confused, but quiet all night; she's been complaining of pain in her foot, especially her toes — in the leg you removed, I mean."

Phantom pain is the strange sensation of discomfort in an extremity that is no longer present. It occurs most commonly in fresh amputees who've had significant pain before their surgery. Unusual for Annie, I thought, because she never complained of pain before the surgery.

"She pulled out her IV once, but we reinserted it. Isn't that right, dear?" she said in an effort to reorient her patient. Annie didn't answer, but when I said, "Good morning," Annie looked at me alertly and said, "Good morning, doctor, how did the operation go?"

The sitter drew her head back, tucked in her chin and said, "She *was* confused!"

"The procedure went well," I said. "As you see, we were able to stay below the knee. We'll have physical therapy come up today for an evaluation. Before you know it, you'll be walking again."

I removed the knee immobilizer; the bandage was a little bloody. That was a good sign. I replaced the knee immobilizer, reassured her, reminded her where the nurse's call button was, and left the room. The sitter followed me out.

"She really was confused," she said, again.

"I know," I said. "White coats will do that; we see it all the time. When the doctor comes in, something clicks. It's a reality check. The confusion disappears, at least temporarily." But Annie's confusion never did return. She remained in the hospital six more days, and then was transferred to a nearby physical rehabilitation facility. They removed her sutures, fitted her for a temporary prosthesis, a pylon, as they are called, and then a permanent prosthesis. Three months later while completing a chart, I looked out my office window and spotted a red-headed lady with red-rimmed glasses, briskly walking the path to my office door.

Bill Murphy, Dialysis Patient

Bill Murphy sat on the wooden bench by his front door. The bus would be out in front in ten minutes. That gave him plenty of time to slip the remaining three socks over his stump and smooth them out. Wrinkles cause big problems. He pulled the plastic mold up over the socks; then he stood up and balanced himself with his left hand on the armrest of the bench. He placed the leg in front of him and planted his stump in the socket. When it felt right, he shifted his weight to that side and pushed down. It slid in all the way. It felt secure. He propped the crutches against the wall by the door. Once the leg was on, he could walk quite normally, without a limp. The articulated ankle joint on his new prosthesis really helped.

The yellow bus pulled up right on time. He saw it pretty well, clearly enough to read the lettering on the side — "Invalid Bus." He climbed in and found his usual seat by Frank, Betty and the other seven riders. He was the last pickup. From here, it was a quick ten-minute shot to the dialysis center. He thought about that word — *invalid*. He resented its hurtful double meaning.

There was a faint odor in the bus, something like a chicken coop, hardly noticeable to him now, after four years. His shift was Tuesday, Thursday and Saturday, 3 to 7 P.M., fifty-two weeks a year. He exited through a side door in the front of the bus. Frank and Betty were helped out, one at a time, through the rear. Their locked wheelchairs fit nicely on the hydraulic lift.

The outpatient dialysis unit was fairly large, but not the biggest in the county. There were two floors, each with two wings. Each wing had 16 recliners, a total of 64 dialysis slots. Each slot contained a large dialysis machine, a bedside table, a small TV suspended from the ceiling, and a blue leather recliner that could be adjusted with the head way down and the feet way up, just in case your blood pressure dropped during the treatment. Bill was in pretty good physical shape, so his slot was on the second floor, in area B. The wheelchair people, visually impaired patients, and shaky people were treated downstairs.

After four years, three sessions a week, he had gotten to know the nurses and aides in his unit pretty well, all of them by their first names. His favorite nurse was Mercedes, but he couldn't count on her being there each time. Mercedes was a good dialysis nurse. She'd knot the rubber tourniquet around his biceps, prep his arm with Betadine and, as if loading a double-barrel shotgun, slide the 16 gauge needles through the skin on his forearm straight into that big bulging vein, the one the surgeon created for him by connecting it to an artery. She never missed. Then he'd settle back, Mercedes would swing the little suspended TV down in front of him, he'd close his eyes, listen to CNN, and rest.

He had been a chef, self-trained, till the diabetes got the best of him. Then his foot went bad. He worked for a while, about five months, with his foot bandaged and covered with a black orthopedic booty with Velcro straps, the one the podiatrist gave him. He started missing work — the standing and all. One night before work, he took his insulin, but he didn't feel like eating. His blood sugar dropped. He sat down dazed and sweating in the corner of the kitchen at the back of the diner. Mr. Karpinos, the manager, called an ambulance. After that, they hired a new night chef. Bill knew they wanted him out of there. That foot had no place in a kitchen.

So now his life was the diabetes, or rather taking care of the complications. Dialysis, he thought, was like having a full-time job anyway. Sometimes he felt real good the next day — sometimes he'd feel all wrung out. Those were the days, he suspected, that they took off too much water. They weighed him before and after each treatment, so he could tell, more or less, how much water they removed.

Aside from June Grasso, the only other dialysis patient Bill knew better than just by name was in the chair to his left. That was Ed. He, too, had end-stage kidney failure from diabetes. He, too, couldn't really see the picture on the little TV. When he was healthy, Ed worked as a builder, houses out in South Jersey. Ed didn't talk much. He was always dozing, his mouth open, his eyes closed, the left one patched. Bill looked at Ed and thought, *He's the house now — vacant, windows boarded, utilities turned off.*

Six years ago, Ed caught a lucky break and got a transplant from his brother, but the kidney died after four years. Ed didn't say why, but Mercedes said he got careless and stopped taking his pills, the immuno-suppressive medication. They didn't talk about it.

During every treatment, someone from the nephrology group, one of the kidney doctors, came to the unit to make rounds. Bill's nephrologist, Dr. Weiss, was young and thorough. Bill knew he could talk to him. Dr. Weiss wasn't full of himself like some of the others. So Bill asked him a question, something he was curious about. "Dr. Weiss," he said, "there are 64 dialysis chairs in this place. How many are filled by diabetics?"

Dr. Weiss corrected him. "Actually, there are 64 chairs, but there are three shifts each day. That's 192 patients per day. The unit is open six days a week ... so, one hundred ninety-two patients each Tuesday, Thursday and Saturday, and an additional hundred ninety-two patients each Monday, Wednesday, and Friday. That's 384 patients," he said.

Then he added, "A few get new kidneys and some move away." (He didn't say some die.) "So the number of diabetics isn't always the same, but I'll find out. I'll let you know next week. There is one thing I can tell you, though. If you look around the unit you'll see that some people are here year after year. I have some diabetic patients who've been on dialysis for over twenty years; they started when I was in high school. Others start, but then seem to get one complication after the next. New research has shown what we suspected all along. That diabetics who control their glucose levels using the HbA1c as a guide have fewer infections and fewer cardiac problems. They survive longer on dialysis."[2]

The following Tuesday, Dr. Weiss had the answer. "Right now," he said, "there are 219 diabetics in this unit, but we have a waiting list."

Bill turned the little TV off and looked around the room. No one's curtains were drawn. The nurses have to keep an eye on everyone, and on the flashing numbers on their dialysis machines. He knew from four years of observation, four hours at a time, three days a week, that the diabetics were often the ones with bandaged feet or eye patches. He knew a little better, now, why they disappeared from time to time. He looked at June Grasso's empty chair and wondered.

Actually, Bill Murphy and Mrs. Grasso were not typical dialysis patients. They managed to avoid being hospitalized for years at a time. On average, according to the statistics in our hospital, chronic outpatient dialysis patients are hospitalized for twelve to fourteen days each year. And according to U.S. dialysis statistics, 20 percent, one in five U.S. dialysis patients, die each year. In the United States today almost half a million people with chronic kidney failure are treated in approximately 5,000 outpatient dialysis facilities.[3] In addition, there are many acute-care in-hospital dialysis units. Because kidney disease in diabetics is progressive and nonreversible, and only 1,521 patients (2006, U.S.A.) receive kidney transplants each year, the diabetic on dialysis remains on dialysis for life.[4]

Nondiabetic patients are a different story. There are instances where their kidney failure can be reversible, cured. The kidneys are sensitive organs. They react to massive bodily stress by shutting down. In patients suffering acute shock resulting from excessive blood loss, for instance, or overwhelming bacterial sepsis (bloodstream infection), a process called acute tubular necrosis (ATN) may occur. In these cases, a short series of dialysis treatments over days or weeks may provide enough time for the patient's own kidneys to recover and produce urine again. Then dialysis can be stopped.

The first successful hemodialysis treatment was administered by Dr. Willem Kolff in the Netherlands in 1945. The patient was not a diabetic; she was treated continually for one week. That was long enough to let her kidneys heal and start working again. The idea of an artificial kidney, and knowledge of the physical principles required to make the machine, took shape slowly during the one hundred years prior to that first treatment. The Scottish chemist Thomas Graham is known as The Father of Diffusion. He was the first, in 1829, to use the principle of diffusion (separation of dissolved substances from water) in the chemistry laboratory. Mr. Graham was not a physician; his interests were rooted purely in chemistry. During his diffusion experiments he used an apparatus which he called a Dialyzer. The word "dialysis" stuck. It was later appropriately applied to the medical process of cleansing blood employing Graham's laws of diffusion.

In 1855, Adolph Fick, a German physiologist, published a description of the diffusion process, but it was Albert Einstein in 1905 who is credited with explaining the scientific underpinning of the diffusion process.[5]

The key component of Dr. Kolff's original dialysis machine was the semi-permeable membrane. Through that membrane, that filter, the first kidney failure patient's blood was cleansed. It was a new product, actually intended for use in the kitchen. It was cellophane — food wrap! Today's sophisticated dialysis machines use complex configurations of synthetic polymers arranged to increase the dialyzing surface. Steadily improving technology allows many chronic dialysis patients to survive for decades while spending only twelve hours per week attached to the machine. But while they are off the machine, sustaining life requires a special low-protein, low-potassium diet and a handful of daily medications.

Today almost half a million people in the United States are on chronic, outpatient hemodialysis. Patients with end-stage, diabetic kidney failure comprise most of this group. The goal of each dialysis treatment is to rid the patient of nitrogenous waste products, excess potassium, and excess water (the patient does not urinate), and to control the tendency to become anemic. All kidney failure patients become anemic. Anemia in hemodialysis patients is treated with oral iron supplements, blood transfusions and the administration of bone marrow-stimulating drugs. These treatments are usually given during the dialysis treatment. Occasionally, life-threatening events such as bleeding or swings in blood pressure occur during dialysis. Experienced dialysis nurses can handle most of these problems, but a physician on the premises would be ideal.

Some outpatient dialysis centers are owned and run by physicians. Large hospitals frequently have their own outpatient dialysis units. They are usually attached or a short distance from the hospital, and they are staffed by the hospital's nephrologists. The majority of outpatient dialysis units, however, are owned by private paramedical companies. Most of these commercial dialysis centers are located in the southern U.S., where obesity and diabetes are rampant. This is a lucrative business. The medical care provided by these private companies may be below par because they are frequently staffed by paramedical personnel, not by physicians.

It is no secret that commercialism in medicine poses a threat to proper medical care. According to Dr. Garabed Eknoyan, president of the National Kidney Foundation, American dialysis patients do not survive as long as Western European or Japanese patients because they may be under-treated or over-treated in order to reach financial goals. Most American dialysis centers operate for profit. This encourages cost-cutting by reusing disposable equipment, shortening treatment sessions to fit in more patients, under-training staff, and functioning without a physician on board. American dialysis patients are either unaware that longer treatments result in longer survival, or, as some believe, are less inclined to sit for longer sessions.[6]

The problem of commercialism in the dialysis unit was recently pointed out in an article in *The New York Times* (*the* "medical journal" for many New York area physicians).[7] It reported that the largest commercial dialysis company in the U.S., Da Vita, is being criticized for possibly jeopardizing the health of its clients by over-using Epogen, the drug most commonly used to treat the chronic anemia of kidney failure. Anemia, a low hemoglobin level, is a constant manifestation of kidney failure. Epogen is an artificial version of erythropoietin, the bone marrow-stimulating hormone produced by normal kidneys. Da Vita's outpatient dialysis clients have been found to have dangerously high hemoglobin levels, indicating the probable over use of Epogen. Da Vita collects more from insurers, primarily Medicare, than it pays Amgen, the manufacturer of the drug. This is but one example of the "profit over patient care" attitude in the U.S. healthcare system — just one more instance of taking money from sick people while risking their health — and this attitude is probably a major reason that the United States is ranked 37th in healthcare systems among all nations by the World Health Organization.[8]

Cutting-edge medical technology has its sneaky side, too. Some doctors and hospitals attract patients under the guise of "progress" — advertising use of the latest medical breakthrough. The introduction of minimally invasive surgery is one example of misused medical progress. This method of surgery is quite appropriate for most gallbladder and GYN procedures. But sometimes minimally invasive surgery is *minimally ethical.*

Consider the plight of the anxious kidney donor. He truly wants to give one of his healthy kidneys to his long suffering brother, a dialysis patient. He's a genetic match, but the thought of major surgery is daunting. He fears big surgery. The surgeon offers to do the procedure laparoscopically. "Well, I can do it through tiny incisions, using a camera and laparoscopic instruments. I operate through tiny tubes, no bigger than straws."

The benevolent but ill-informed kidney donor assumes he'll benefit from state-of-the-art medical technology. He is unaware that his avocado-sized kidney will not fit through that laparoscopic bullet-hole beneath his belly button. Nor is he aware that donating his kidney the old-fashioned way through a six- or seven-inch incision is safer, with hands-on technique, and takes less than an hour. Whereas the laparoscopic technique of kidney removal may take many hours, (four or five is not unusual) and the laparoscopic technique carries significant risks of its own. The last step of the laparoscopic procedure is to extract that kidney from the donor's belly. To get it out, the surgeon must make an incision — an incision almost as long as the one used with the open, faster, and safer old-fashioned technique. If I ever need to donate a kidney, it'll be the old-fashioned way.

According to my observations, the most common reasons for inadequate dialysis treatments are:

(1) A poorly functioning dialysis fistula or catheter, which provides too little blood-flow from the patient to the dialysis machine. Each dialysis machine provides a readout indicating the number of milliliters of blood flowing through the machine per minute. A good functioning fistula or dialysis catheter will yield 300 or more milliliters per minute.

(2) An inadequate duration of treatment. Each treatment should last at least 4 hours (some centers cut treatments short). Shorter treatments are less effective.

(3) A misjudged quantity of water removed. The removal of too little water (remember, most dialysis patients don't urinate) may result in shortness of breath or heart failure. The removal of too much water may result in weakness, dehydration or a sudden drop in blood pressure.

Perhaps these are some of the reasons that dialysis patients treated in the United States die at nearly twice the rate of dialysis patients in Europe and Japan.

In the United States, the majority of the nearly half-million dialysis patients receive treatment in a hospital or in an outpatient dialysis unit. An additional 2,000 or so receive their hemodialysis at home, either because they can afford to do so or because they are too ill to be transported. The remaining 30,000 kidney failure patients are kept alive by an entirely different process, *peritoneal dialysis*.

Peritoneal Dialysis

The inner lining of the entire abdominal cavity and the outer coat of all the intra-abdominal organs, liver, spleen, large and small intestines, etc., is composed of a membrane, much like the skin of a hot dog. This membrane, the peritoneal lining, is only one cell thick; it's smooth, slippery and slightly wet. When bathed in hypertonic dialysis solution, the peritoneum becomes a semi-permeable membrane, like the cellophane used in that very first dialysis treatment. Dialysis solution, when instilled into the abdomen, draws potassium, excess body fluids and nitrogenous waste through the peritoneum and into the solution. Thus, a patient's own peritoneum is converted, with some inconvenience, into an artificial kidney. An alternative to hemodialysis, the process is called *peritoneal dialysis*.

Peritoneal dialysis requires active patient participation. It works best for motivated patients. As with hemodialysis, peritoneal dialysis requires surgical preparation — the operative placement of a flexible, pencil-sized, clear Teflon tube through the skin and muscular abdominal wall. The tube serves as a conduit for passage of the dialisate solution into and out of the abdominal cavity. The tube is equipped with two, Velcro-like cuffs which, when placed above and below the rectus muscle, become solidly scarred in so the tube, called a Tenkoff catheter, will not fall out.

Whereas hemodialysis is required three times per week, peritoneal dialysis is performed daily, usually overnight, so the patient has the daytime free. The dialisate solution is delivered to the patient's house by a medical supply company. It arrives in plastic bags that are similar to, but much larger than, IV bags. The bags are hung on a pole; sterile tubing connects the bag to the abdominal catheter, and gravity pulls the fluid into the abdominal cavity. The fluid remains in the abdomen for a prescribed length of time (the dwell time); then the plastic bag is placed on the floor, allowing gravity to siphon the waste-laden fluid out of the abdomen and back into the bag. The process is repeated four to six times (these are called exchanges). A machine called a cycler, which allows the patient to self-administer the treatment while he sleeps through the night, can facilitate the process.

The advantage of peritoneal dialysis is that after one or two training sessions with a dialysis nurse, it can be done at home with little or no assistance from a family member or healthcare professional. The nephrologist sets the quantity and strength of dialysis solution to be used, the dwell time, and the frequency of the treatments. These parameters are based on blood test results that reflect the effectiveness of the first few hospital-administered treatments. Since peritoneal dialysis works by osmosis and diffusion, the amount of water removed can be adjusted by increasing or decreasing the osmolarity of the dialisate solution, or by adjusting the dwell time of the solution.

The major disadvantages of peritoneal dialysis are the need for daily treatments, the discomfort of a catheter protruding from the belly, and the constant threat of infection from the catheter, as it connects the inside of the abdomen to the outside world. The surgical procedure required to insert the peritoneal dialysis catheter is usually done under general anesthesia, but local anesthesia with sedation is an option for the stoic patient. The Tenkoff catheter is placed so that it exits the abdomen slightly below and to the left of the belly button. The portion of the catheter that lies within the abdominal cavity is directed into the pelvic area, because that's where most of the fluid collects. The catheter is positioned such that each of its two, Velcro-like cuffs sit above and below the rectus muscle. These cuffs form an adherent scar with the surrounding tissue; this fixes the catheter in place. Once healed, it's like another extremity; it cannot be pulled out. Removal requires another trip to the operating room. Ideally, the catheter should be placed in the abdomen several weeks prior to the start of treatments so that it scars in tightly before the treatments begin.

Chapter 9

CAROTID ARTERY DISEASE AND STROKE: THE CASE OF MR. CROWE

Mr. Crowe was a 68-year-old lawyer from Hoboken. He was an insulin-controlled, type 2 diabetic with mild hypertension. I'd met him and his wife, Betty, a week earlier in my office. According to Betty, her husband took good care of his diabetes, that is his blood sugar, but he ignored his high blood pressure. That was a mistake.

I didn't know who had referred him. When I asked, he simply said, "A nurse." He'd already seen an ophthalmologist and had undergone an ultrasound examination of his carotid arteries in our hospital's vascular laboratory.

His problem started one evening while he was eating dinner. He experienced a sudden episode of partial blindness in his right eye. It lasted about thirty minutes. When it happened, Betty left the dishes on the table and took him directly to the emergency room, but by the time they got there, his vision had returned. The E.R. receptionist told him he'd see the triage nurse shortly and sat him in the waiting room. Thirty-five minutes went by, but no one approached him. The waiting room was full. He became impatient and left. Betty, annoyed at him for walking out, insisted on driving home.

He was okay for a week, but then the same thing happened again in the same eye. This time it happened during breakfast — it was as if a shade had been drawn halfway down over the eye. Betty called her eye doctor. He told them to come right over. But by the time the Crowes got there, the problem, once again, was gone; her husband was seeing quite normally.

It was early. He was the first patient in the ophthalmologist's office that morning. The doctor, having obtained a brief history over the phone, looked his patient over. He had Mr. Crowe follow his finger up and down and side to side. Then he removed Mr. Crowe's glasses. He put some drops in both eyes to dilate the pupils; then he leaned forward and, nose to nose, placed his ophthalmoscope between his eye and Mr. Crowe's right eye. He looked for half a minute or so, and then he looked into the left eye.

He pushed himself back on the rolling chair and said, "You've had a mini stroke. Two mini strokes." He went on to explain that a tiny piece of atherosclerotic plaque had apparently broken off the lining of the main artery in his neck, his carotid artery. The fleck of plaque was then carried by the flowing blood up towards his brain, but before it could get there, it veered into his right ophthalmic artery, the artery to his right eye. The tiny particle then lodged in a small retinal vessel causing it to close off in temporary spasm. The lack of blood flow to part of the retina caused the episodes of partial blindness. When the spasm subsided, the blood supply was replenished and Mr. Crowe's vision returned.

The pieces of plaque were still there. The doctor could see them lying in the small translucent retinal arteries, like little pieces of amber. "They're called Hollenhorst plaques," he said. "You've had what is called *amorosis fugax*. If that fleck of plaque was larger, you would have had an ocular stroke — permanent blindness in that eye. If the plaque had floated up past your opthalmic artery into your brain, you would have had different symptoms. It's serious. You have to see a vascular surgeon."

Another name for a mini stroke is a transient ischemic attack (TIA). It's a warning sign, an indication of an impending permanent stroke. Mini strokes last minutes or hours. They can cause temporary blindness, as with Mr. Crowe, or temporary paralysis of an arm or a leg, or both, or a brief inability to speak. A mini stroke that lasts longer, up to a week, is called a resolving neurologic deficit (RIND). If the neurological problem remains longer than that, it's an outright stroke.

A sudden temporary loss of consciousness, fainting, is often mistaken for a mini stroke. But fainting is usually not a purely neurological event. Doctors refer to fainting as a *vagal reaction* because the vagus nerve plays a role in blood pressure regulation. From time to time we see vagal reactions in the office. They may be triggered simply by the sight of blood, or, in the elderly, by a sudden change to the upright position.

How Do You Pick a Surgeon?

"You know any surgeons?" the ophthalmologist asked.

"Yes, Dr. Small. He repaired my hernia. He was very good. I'll call him."

"Is he a vascular surgeon?" the eye doctor asked.

"I don't think so; the sign on his door says 'General Surgery.'"

"You need a vascular surgeon, a surgeon who deals with blood vessels. Stop at the desk. My nurse will give you a list of vascular surgeons. It's important that you do it right away. The next episode may be a full-blown stroke!"

Betty took him by the hand and they left the office. They sat in the car for a few moments, examining the list of vascular surgeons. They chose one at random, Dr. Troop. When they got home, they looked him up to see if he participated in their HMO. He did. They arranged an appointment for the following afternoon.

Dr. Troop was tall. He had a neatly trimmed mustache and wore a vest to match his suit. Betty noticed the many diplomas on his wall. He'd graduated from medical school in New York City, completed his surgical residency at the same hospital center, and did his vascular training in The Bronx. Dr. Troop ushered them into his examining room, and, in a deep, authoritative voice, asked Mr. Crowe to unbutton the collar of his shirt. Then he took his stethoscope, which had been draped around his neck, plugged it in his ears and placed the cold metal against Mr. Crowe's neck. First he listened on the right side, then on the left, then again on the right. He was listening for a bruit, that abnormal whistling sound indicative of a narrowed blood vessel, the carotid artery in this case. "You have a bruit on the right side," he said, and explained again what the ophthalmologist had said, that the rapid flow of blood through that narrow spot in the carotid artery had likely knocked off some small pieces of plaque, which then lodged in Mr. Crowe's ophthalmic artery, the artery to his eye. This caused temporary blindness.

The Crowes sat in Dr. Troop's consultation room and listened to a long-winded explanation of carotid artery disease, the crux of which was that Mr. Crowe needed an ultrasound, a Doppler examination of his carotid arteries. Pending the result, he would probably need an operation to clear the artery of plaque and keep him from having a major stroke. Dr. Troop gave Mr. Crowe a prescription for the ultrasound exam. Then he asked his nurse to arrange it for the following morning.

Lillian, the ultrasound tech, was middle-aged, serious and very professional. She had worked in the vascular lab for seven years. She was very adept. She had Mr. Crowe lie flat on the examining table, placed his shirt on the hook in the corner of the room and turned on the ultrasound machine. Then she explained the procedure. "We'll start on the right," she said. "I need you to turn your head to the left." From a squeeze bottle, she squirted some warm jelly over the right side of his neck. Then she took the ultrasound probe, which looked like his electric shaver, and placed it in the jelly. She pressed lightly as she slid the probe up and down his neck. As she moved it, she watched the screen on the ultrasound monitor. They could hear the sound of the blood flowing through Mr. Crowe's carotid artery, a pulsating swish — lull — swish — lull. She turned the volume down. She moved the probe towards the back of his neck and repeated the procedure. Then she wiped the jelly off, had him turn his head to the right, squirted some jelly on the left side of his neck and did the whole thing again.

She typed up the data on the keyboard of the ultrasound machine as the test progressed. Then she wiped the jelly off. "Done," she said, and took his hand to help him sit up. She handed Mr. Crowe his shirt.

"Well, that was easy," Mr. Crowe said. "What did you find?"

"There are some changes," she said. "But I'm not permitted to tell you what the findings are. I'll call your doctor; he's responsible for the final reading. Oh!" Lillian had glanced at Dr. Troop's name on the prescription in her hand.

"Is something wrong?" Mr. Crowe said.

"Ha ... have you known Dr. Troop long?" Lillian asked, with a tilt of her head.

"No, I only met him that one time in the office."

"Well, I'll fax him a copy of the ultrasound results. You give him a call; he'll explain the findings. Good luck. It was nice meeting you." She shook his hand and left the room.

Mr. Crowe put on his shirt, scratched his head, and went to the waiting area to find Betty. "You look upset," she said. "What did they find? Do you need an operation?"

"Come on let's go. I'll tell you in the car." As they walked towards the door, he glanced back. No Lillian. "I don't know what the test showed," he said, "but I got the feeling that the ultrasound lady didn't think much of Dr. Troop."

"Why do you say that?" Betty asked.

"Well, you remember when I had my hernia repaired, how all the nurses spoke so highly of Dr. Small?"

"Yes," Betty said. "But what does that have to do with the test?"

"Well, nothing, but the ultrasound lady didn't say a word about Dr. Troop."

"Maybe she doesn't know him."

"How could she not know him? This is the vascular lab, and he's a vascular surgeon."

"Maybe she's not supposed to say anything," Betty said.

"No ... no ... I definitely picked up some bad vibes. I'm going to call Dr. Small. I'll see who he suggests."

During that first office visit with Mr. Crowe, I went over his history: the two episodes of temporary blindness, his trip to the ophthalmologist, and the visit to the vascular lab. He didn't mention Dr. Troop or how he got my name. I noticed Troop's name, though, as the referring doctor on the ultrasound report. I said nothing. I knew that Dr. Troop gave the illusion of competence. I knew, too, that as soon as his patients said "Troop" to a nurse — any nurse — the illusion would vanish. A surgeon's reputation is a part of his hospital, like the bricks and mortar. Reputations are not always fair. In Troop's case, though, it was right on target.

The ultrasound report showed a 90 percent occlusion of the proximal right internal carotid artery. Mr. Crowe needed the most common major operative procedure performed by vascular surgeons, a carotid endarterectomy. He knew the answer, but Mr. Crowe asked the question anyway. "What if I don't have the surgery? What if I just take blood thinners?"

I gave him the facts. "Well, if the artery closes completely, you have a 50–50 chance of having a stroke on the spot. You've already proven that you have unstable plaque in your carotid artery. Pieces have already broken off. They were tiny pieces, but if a large piece of plaque comes off, it will lodge in your brain and cause a major stroke. The operation itself carries a stroke risk too, about 2 percent. But the chances of your having a stroke without the surgery are much, much greater. You need the operation."

Then, as often happens, he wanted the surgery right away. I told him it should be done soon, but first he'd need a baseline CAT scan of his brain and approval from his cardiologist. Diabetics, indeed, anyone with a major arterial blockage in one place, may have a blockage elsewhere. I called Gail into the consultation room. The three of us went over the preoperative workup, the blood work, coagulation profile, chest X-ray, and the CAT scan of his brain. I told Mr. Crowe we would leave the EKG for the cardiologist. "Gail will call with an operative date," I said, "and because you're taking insulin, we'll arrange for your operation to be done first thing in the morning. I'll coordinate everything with your diabetologist. He may want to admit you the night before. You can't eat for eight hours prior to the surgery, so he'll want to adjust your insulin dose. You'll probably be placed on an insulin drip. We'll get you done before the end of the week."

Mr. Crowe's Carotid Endarterectomy

To this point, the day of the surgery, everything had worked out as planned. Mr. Crowe was admitted the night before, started on an insulin drip, and cleared by his cardiologist, and the blood work and CAT scan were completely normal.

I went down to the surgical holding area, where the paperwork is reviewed and the preoperative patients are checked, gowned, and asked to sign a consent form before they are wheeled into the operating room. I found the anesthesiologist, Dr. Jane Randall, sitting with Mr. Crowe. She was explaining that his operation would be delayed, "bumped" by another surgeon's emergency. I said hello to Mr. Crowe. I'd seen him on rounds the previous night and obtained the surgical consent. I motioned Dr. Randall aside and asked her what the problem was.

She whispered, "Dr. Troop had an emergency. He had to take his patient from yesterday evening back into surgery. He was bleeding into the neck incision."

"Why didn't he take him back last night?" I inquired.

"I guess he thought it would stop," she said.

"There are 23 operating rooms. Why did they take ours?"

"Yours was the only one set up for a vascular procedure, and he needed the room right away. He's fast. He should be out of there soon."

Each of us knew what the other was thinking. This was a recurring event. The reason Dr. Troop needed to take the patient back was precisely because he was fast. Too fast. He, like many busy surgeons, confused speed with good surgery. When you do that, you cannot be meticulous, and meticulous surgeons have fewer complications. Dr. Troop is no slouch. He's intelligent, well trained, and totally involved with his work, but too often his postoperative patients bleed or leak or develop some other unexpected problem that demands a quick return to the operating room. Troop was Albert Einstein on rounds, but Jackson Pollock in the O.R. His nickname, "the comeback kid," was well earned.

I told Mr. Crowe that I would get to him as soon as possible. I paged the third-year surgical resident, my scheduled assistant, to tell him we were bumped. Now I had time to finish rounds and have breakfast.

Waiting for O.R. Time

Surgeons spend a lot of time waiting. Operating rooms are never on schedule. We have to use that time effectively. I usually make rounds or go to the record room to complete charts. Rounds went quickly. My first stop is usually the ICU. Mr. Collins, my post-op pancreatic resection, was ready for transfer. His incision was clean, he had passed some gas and his jaundice was almost gone. I removed his nasogastric tube, started him on sips of fluids and discussed the transfer orders with the ICU resident. Next, I saw Mrs. Findlay; she was four days post bowel resection for perforated diverticulitis. I advanced her diet, checked her wound, and reviewed her blood work.

Then I saw Mr. Daley, a 46-year-old cartoonist. He was a type 2, insulin-requiring diabetic. He'd come in via the emergency room a week earlier with a badly infected left great toe. Somehow, he had stepped on one of his insulin needles and broken it off at the hub, and with his neuropathy, he never felt a thing. He walked with the needle in his toe for days, maybe weeks, before his wife noticed the blood on his sock. She looked at his foot. It was red and swollen. She spotted a pinhole opening in the meaty part of his big toe. She took him to the E.R. where X-rays showed the broken needle deep under the skin. The X-ray also revealed the not-so-subtle appearance of osteomyelitis, a bone infection. It takes a few weeks for the bony changes of osteomyelitis to show up on an X-ray, so he probably was walking around on that needle for quite some time.

Back in the 1970s, when shag rugs were popular, we saw a lot of feet with embedded needles. I asked his wife if they had a shag rug. She looked at me and said, "Yes. Why ... how did you know that?" I explained that when a needle falls on a shag rug, it often stays upright. If the rug is flat, with no pile, like an Oriental rug, the needle lies flat and even if you step on it, it won't penetrate the skin.

That night in the E.R., I removed the needle through a small incision.

I drained the abscess, cultured the pus, and packed the wound with a small piece of damp gauze. I checked Mr. Daley's circulation. It was excellent. He had bounding pulses in both feet. His white blood count was 12,000, slightly elevated, consistent with his infection. His creatinine was 1.6, indicating he had mildly impaired kidney function. But Mr. Daley had severe, advanced osteomyelitis in a distal bone of the toe. In my experience, that will not respond to antibiotics.

I called the people in the infectious disease service for their input. In my mind, there was no question; the toe needed to be removed. But I'd just met Mr. Daley. I wanted him to hear the news from a non-surgeon as well. Unfortunately, the infectious disease doctor thought differently. He suggested that I insert a central intravenous line. That is, he wanted me to place a catheter in Mr. Daley's internal jugular or subclavian vein for the administration of six weeks of intensive antibiotic therapy.

I rarely disagree with a physician after I have called him in for consultation, but I disagreed with this doctor. First, the very act of placing the central intravenous line carries minimal but real risks of pneumothorax (puncture of the lung), as well as bleeding, and even a bloodstream infection from the longterm presence of the intravenous line itself. The IV line forms a path directly from the skin to the bloodstream. And secondly, six weeks of intravenous antibiotics carries significant risks of its own. One of the most common problems associated with longterm antibiotic therapy is the development of a "C-Diff" (clostridium difficile) infection, *pseudomembranous enterocolitis.* This is a severe infection of the lower gastrointestinal tract. It occurs when the antibiotic used to fight the infection kills the natural protective bacterial flora in the patient's large intestine as well. This opens the door for a pathological bacterium to colonize the colon. Patients with C-diff experience severe watery diarrhea, fever, and damage to the wall of the large intestine. Perforation of the colon occurs in rare cases. The treatment for C-Diff involves giving more antibiotics (usually vancomycin by mouth) and if the infection persists, then extensive surgery is required to remove the damaged bowel. Pseudomembranous enterocolitis is one of the most common hospital-acquired (nosocomial) infections in the United States. At any given time, in any given hospital, you will find several cases of this difficult to treat, sometimes fatal hospital-acquired infection. Longterm antibiotics have their place, but not in Mr. Daley's case.

Then, of course, there is the ever present risk of MRSA, methacillin resistant Staphylococcus Aureus, perhaps the most notorious, potentially fatal hospital-acquired infection. According to the *Guardian Unlimited* of Portsmouth, in the U.K., this infection is so common in Europe that some would-be hospital patients refuse admission for fear of acquiring it. All of these infections are, in great part, the result of physicians' injudicious overuse of antibiotics.

Mr. Daley needed an explanation. I know that, given a choice, most patients will choose non-operative treatment over a surgical procedure. I sat down with him and explained my view regarding the use of longterm antibiotics for osteomyelitis of the toe. I explained that each specialist tends to treat a given disease using the methods familiar to his own area of expertise. We went over the limitations imposed by his mild kidney dysfunction, the risks of central venous line insertions, and the possibility of contracting a hospital acquired infection. I told him that I felt the best treatment for him, in view of his good circulation and the probability of normal healing, would be a toe amputation. I expected a flat refusal, or at least an argument. I got neither.

"I can live with that," he said. "All my cartoon characters do. They all have four fingers and toes. Most people don't notice," he said, "but from the beginning, cartoon characters were drawn with four fingers and four toes, because it saves time. And even now, with digital animation techniques, they still have four fingers and toes."

I placed him on preoperative IV antibiotics, and two days later, when the soft tissue swelling had subsided, I amputated his toe. His lack of pain sensation, the neuropathy, spared him the need for and the risks of anesthesia. I removed the metatarsal head, the bony prominence forming the ball joint of that toe, as well. This would eliminate the occurrence of ulceration over a bony, insensate (numb) pressure point, and give his foot a more streamlined appearance. With a proper fitting shoe, he would walk without a limp.

I examined his foot. There were no signs of infection. The nylon sutures would remain in place for another eight to ten days. I placed a wraparound bandage held on with flexible netting. No tape. I told him to keep it dry, elevate the foot of his bed, and keep his walking to a minimum. I discharged him without a prescription for antibiotics. He didn't need them because the infected bone was in a specimen bottle now, and his blood cultures had never been positive. I told him to call my office for a follow-up appointment.

There's an old surgical expression — "the best post-operative care is a good operation." In other words, if the surgeon does the operation well, then the post-operative course will be uncomplicated. It's true, most of the time but detailed postoperative care is as important as the surgery itself. Too often in today's medical world, a significant part of a patient's post-op care is relegated to house staff or a surgeon's partners; people who were not present during the surgery. No one is as well-equipped or as motivated to assure a smooth post-op course as the surgeon who did the surgery. So how do you pick a surgeon? You ask the opinion of an O.R. nurse if you're lucky enough to know one, one who's been around for a while. Anyone else's opinion is suspect.

Finished with rounds, I went to the cafeteria for breakfast. I found the third-year resident sitting at a table in the corner of the doctor's area.

"Have you had a chance to look at Mr. Crowe's carotid ultrasound?" I asked.

"No, but I have a copy of his report here." He pulled a folded white sheet from his lab coat pocket and flattened it on the cafeteria table. "Looks like he's got a pretty high-grade stenosis; 90 percent on the right. The left carotid artery is clean, though, and both vertebrals are open."

Just then, the third-year medical student assigned to our team wandered into the cafeteria. We motioned him over.

"Are you scrubbing on this carotid?" the resident asked.

"I'd like to," the student said, "but I have a lecture at noon."

"That's okay," the resident said. "We'll get you out by then. Take a look at this report." He slid the ultrasound report in front of the student. "What do you think?"

The student had never seen a carotid ultrasound report. "Well," he said. "It looks like there's a blockage right here." He pointed to the black, hourglass-shaped ink mark in the right carotid artery.

"What's the significance of that?" the resident asked.

"Well if it closes, he'll get a stroke."

The resident responded, "Well he's already had two TIAs. How do you account for that?"

The medical student hesitated. "Not enough blood getting through?"

The resident enlightened him. "First of all, you know what a TIA is, right?"

"Yeah, it's a mini stroke."

"That's right," the resident said. "In his case, the mini stroke took the form of temporary blindness in his right eye, but it wasn't because of the narrowing itself. It was because a piece of the plaque that was causing the narrowing broke off and lodged in the artery supplying blood to his right eye. Remember your anatomy? Everyone has four arteries supplying blood to his brain, the two vertebrals in the back of the neck, and the two carotids in the front. They join in the middle of the brain, forming that circular vessel, the Circle of Willis. Some people can develop 100 percent blockage of a carotid artery and still not have a stroke. That's because the arteries in the brain are all connected, sort of like a spider web; it's a natural protective mechanism."

I interjected, "There's a 50–50 chance of getting a stroke, if you develop a complete blockage of a carotid artery. It doesn't matter whether the artery is tied off intentionally during an operative procedure, say for removal of a tumor, or if it closes from atherosclerosis. Most strokes, however, are the result of pieces of atherosclerotic plaque or a clot breaking off from the narrowed area and sailing up into the brain with the flow of blood.

"I have two physician-patients with carotid artery disease who are on the staff here. One, a hematologist, has one carotid closed and the other 50 percent narrowed, and the other doctor, a family practitioner, has both carotids completely closed. Both doctors are functioning normally, and neither has had a stroke or TIA. The hematologist has been a latent type 1 diabetic (LADA) for almost 50 years. The family practitioner isn't a diabetic, but he's still a heavy smoker."

"Why don't you fix it? The obstruction I mean," the student asked.

"Because, once the carotid artery is completely, that is 100 percent, blocked, whether it's symptomatic or not, operating on it can only make it worse. The general guideline is: if the patient has a greater than 75 percent carotid artery blockage, then surgery, carotid endarterectomy, should be done, because without the surgery the stroke rate is extremely high. Once the artery is 100 percent closed, though, no surgery should be done."

"What about carotid stunts?" the student asked.

"You mean *stents*," I said. "Carotid stents are good in certain situations, with extreme narrowing due to scarring from radiation treatment, for example, but in general, they are just what you said, 'stunts.' The procedure has a significantly higher stroke rate than traditional open carotid endarterectomy. That's because the stent must be pushed through the narrowed area before it's deployed and that can dislodge plaque, which can cause a stroke."

My cell phone rang; it was Sue in the O.R. "We're ready. They're wheeling Mr. Crowe into room nine. Come on up."

The three of us went up to the locker room, changed into scrubs, put on our caps and masks and entered O.R. number nine.

Mr. Crowe was already on the table. Dr. Randall had started an IV in his right arm and was busy placing an arterial line into his radial artery, in the left wrist. I explained to the student that the arterial line, when hooked up to the monitor, will give the anesthesiologist a continual readout of Mr. Crowe's blood pressure. Blood pressure control is very important during this type of surgery. If it's too high, the patient can bleed into his brain. If it's too low, the artery we're working on can clot. Dr. Randall can control the blood pressure with fast-acting, intravenous drugs.

Carotid Artery Surgery

I always remain in the operating room while the anesthesiologist puts my patient to sleep. Sometimes the anesthesia is more risky than the surgery. Dr. Randall injected her concoction of intravenous medications. Mr. Crowe was quickly asleep and the muscle relaxant had intentionally stopped his breathing. Dr. Randall was assisted by a first-year, female anesthesia resident. She handed the resident the endotracheal tube and said, "Here. Why don't you try the intubation."

I intervened. "No. Not this case. Not on a carotid. You do it." Had it not been a first-year resident, I would've said nothing, but the last thing Mr. Crowe needed was a first-year anesthesia resident struggling to place the endotracheal tube. The oxygen level in his brain is my responsibility.

Dr. Randall places the tube with ease. The third-year resident, the student and I go to the scrub sinks, complete our five-minute scrub, and return, hands dripping. Dorothy, the circulating nurse, helps us with our gowns, and Diane, the scrub nurse, holds our gloves open for us. I direct Dorothy as she repositions Mr. Crowe's head, extending it backwards and facing left. We paint the neck with Betadine, place the sterile towels and drapes. We're ready to start. I lift Mr. Crowe's head and turn it back towards me. This shows me the crease in his neck where I'll make my incision. I mark the crease with a sterile marking pen and turn his head back, away from me.

"I like to make my incisions in skin creases," I tell the student. "That way they'll heal with a hidden scar."

Diane hands me the scalpel. I make my incision through the inked area for a distance of 4 or 5 inches. The neck has a very rich blood supply;

everything bleeds. I stop the bleeding with small clamps and fine silk ties. I use the electrocautery to stop tiny bleeding points. Just beneath the subcutaneous tissue lies the platysma, a wide but very thin sheet of muscle. I transect it using the electrocautery; this exposes the deep fascia of the neck, external jugular vein and occipital nerve. I show the student how to hold the sterno-mastoid muscle out of my way. Then I place a self-retaining retractor in the wound and ratchet it open to hold the incision apart. I clamp, divide and tie off the tissue overlying the internal jugular vein. Then I ligate the facial vein with two 3–0 silk ties. With my scalpel, I divide it, leaving one stump on the blue translucent internal jugular. I realign my tissue retractors and gently push the cigar-sized internal jugular aside. This exposes the pulsating common carotid artery.

Mr. Crowe's problem, the narrowed, plaque-filled segment of carotid artery, is a little higher in the neck. I can't see it yet. It is in the usual spot, where the artery divides into its internal and external branches. I carry my dissection upward towards the ear. I spot the hypoglossal nerve, the nerve to the tongue. I'm careful not to cut it. If I do, his tongue will permanently drift to the left side of his mouth, between his teeth, and he'll bite it constantly. Eating will be difficult. I carefully dissect; exposing the carotid artery up to the base of the skull, where the hypoglossal nerve crosses over it. It is a big nerve, the size of a dandelion stem, but yellow and shiny. I run my finger gently over the anterior surface of the carotid artery. I can feel the obstructing plaque through the pulsating artery wall.

The plaque sits where the artery divides, where it bifurcates into the external branch, which supplies blood to his face and the internal branch, which carries blood to the right side of his brain. The plaque extends up into the internal branch of the carotid artery for half an inch. I feel it through the artery wall, hoping it does not extend beyond my reach. My finger finds a soft spot above plaque. Using narrow, blue latex ribbons, I double-loop each arterial branch: the common carotid artery below the obstructing plaque, and the internal and the external carotid arteries above the plaque. When I pull up on the latex ribbons, the loops close — I can stop the flow of blood to Mr. Crowe's brain. I have control of the carotid artery now.

I expose the vagus nerve. It's five times the size of the hypoglossal. It runs alongside and just beneath the carotid artery. If the vagus nerve is clamped, cut, or caught in the loop of the latex ribbon, it will not function. That would impede Mr. Crowe's swallowing. He'll choke on his food. Not a good thing. I make sure not to injure it. The carotid is totally exposed now, from the root of the neck to the angle of the jaw. We're set, now, to do the operation.

I ask the resident, "Are you ready?"

"For what?" he says.

I hand him the suction.

"Your job is to suck the blood away so I can see to work." I check with Diane. She has all my instruments ready. I look at the heart monitor and check the blood pressure, 140 mm of mercury. I jokingly test the student—"What do I do next?"

He answers, "I don't know. I'm gonna be a pediatrician."

"When you clamp an artery," I tell him, "you must first give an anticoagulant, because non-flowing blood will clot. We don't want a clot in his brain, so we give him a fast-acting anticoagulant, an intravenous bolus of 5,000 units of heparin." I nod to the anesthesiologist. She injects the heparin. We wait a full minute to make sure it's in effect. I tighten the latex ribbon above the plaque in the internal carotid artery and clamp the taut ribbon to the cloth drape by Mr. Crowe's ear. I've cut off the major blood supply to the right side of his brain.

I pull tight on the latex ribbon surrounding the common carotid artery. But the vessel continues to pulsate. There is so much calcium in the walls that it will not close. I slip the jaws of a small vascular clamp, one which will not damage the artery wall, around the vessel and close it. Then I tighten the latex ribbon around the external carotid. I pull up on the silk ties that I've placed around the two small branches of the external carotid, the artery to the tongue (the lingual artery) and the superior thyroid artery. All the branches are closed now; I'm ready to open the carotid artery. Ten seconds pass. Is the right side of the brain getting enough blood?

If all the branches are clamped, there should be no bleeding when I open the vessel. Diane hands me the scalpel; I make a 1 cm incision in the common carotid just below the obstructing plaque. The artery is stiff, heavily calcified. It's hard to cut. I give the scalpel back and take a right angle arterial scissors. I cut through the calcified plaque, continuing up to the soft area of the internal carotid artery just below its latex loop. It's like opening one side of a pea pod and exposing the peas. I irrigate the open area with saline from a syringe with a blunt-tipped needle. I suck the blood and saline out with a small, metal, suction tip. I peek up at the student. "Watch this," I say. Then I loosen the latex loop around the internal carotid artery, letting the blood flow back out of the brain and into the opened artery. I hold the latex loop with my left hand, and use the suction with my right. I quickly pull the loop up again, tightening it like a noose to stop the backflow. "That was nice bleeding; good backflow, almost pulsatile.

"A strong backflow indicates that the right side of the brain is getting enough blood. We don't need to use a shunt."

"What's the difference between a shunt and a stent?" the student asks.

"Stents are permanent springs placed within a vessel. They hold a narrowed segment of artery open. In a minute, I'll show you a shunt."

I continue to work as I speak to the student. "I was testing the backflow, estimating how much blood is coming from the left side of the brain to the right side via the other carotid and the vertebral arteries. If there is a decent backflow, then there should be enough blood flow to the right side of the brain to keep it alive, enough oxygen to avoid a stroke. Just a trickle coming back at us would indicate that the right hemisphere is not getting enough blood. Then, to avoid a stroke during the surgery, I'd have to use a temporary shunt, a thin flexible tube, to carry blood around the clamped artery to the right side of the brain."

Diane dangles the little plastic, hose-like shunt in front of the student's face. "I find it necessary to use a shunt in about one out of ten carotids," I tell him. "Some surgeons shunt every carotid, but shoving that silicone shunt up the artery toward the brain carries its own risks."

Diane hands me a vascular forceps and a small spatulated instrument called an elevator. I begin to remove the obstructing plaque. First, I find the plane, the space between the plaque and the thin, outer layer of the arterial wall, the adventitia. Every artery has a three-layered wall. The outermost layer is the adventitia. It's very thin. You can practically see through it. The middle layer, the media, is where calcium accumulates as we age. This process, calcification, is especially pronounced in diabetics and smokers. In Mr. Crowe's case, as in most diabetics, the media is hard, like an eggshell. The third layer of an artery, the inner lining, is called the intima. The intima is where lipids and cholesterol are deposited as plaque.

Plaque varies in consistency. It can be soft like cottage cheese, firm like cooked egg yoke, or hard like frozen butter. Mr. Crowe's plaque is soft, the kind that breaks off easily. I use delicate forceps and the blunt end of a small clamp to carefully peel it out of the open artery. The plaque feathers off into a razor thin lip at two and a half centimeters up into the internal carotid artery. A part of the plaque extends up into the external branch as well. I carefully pull that part of the plaque out with my forceps, like taking a pimento from an olive. The entire plaque comes out in one, Y-shaped piece; in the center there is a narrow channel where the blood had been coursing through on its way to the brain (figs. 11, 12).

I hand the specimen off to Diane. I use my vascular forceps to carefully peel out the few remaining bits of plaque that cling to the fragile adventitia. I irrigate with saline. Then I momentarily loosen the latex loop around the internal carotid, letting the backflow of blood wash any pieces of loose plaque out of the artery. I back bleed the external carotid as well. Then I ask the intern to step back so he won't get splashed with blood as I open, then quickly close the clamp on the common carotid artery. This gets rid of any clot that may have formed below the clamp. We irrigate with saline and suck the vessel clean. I explain to the student that we could simply sew the vessel closed with fine nylon stitches, but that would narrow the lumen.

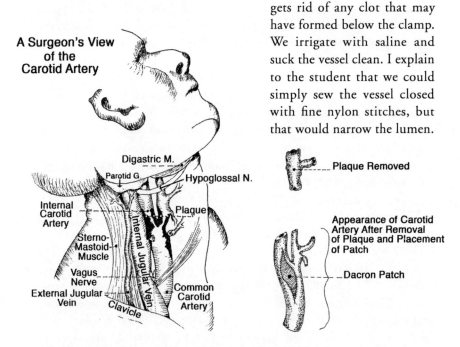

A Surgeon's View of the Carotid Artery

Digastric M.

Parotid G.

Hypoglossal N.

Internal Carotid Artery

Plaque

Sterno-Mastoid Muscle

Internal Jugular Vein

Vagus Nerve

External Jugular Vein

Clavicle

Common Carotid Artery

Plaque Removed

Appearance of Carotid Artery After Removal of Plaque and Placement of Patch

Dacron Patch

Fig. #11 and 12: The anatomy of the carotid artery. Strokes are twice as common in diabetics as in non-diabetics. Carotid endarterectomy is the operation designed to prevent strokes. Most strokes are the result of plaque buildup in the carotid arteries. The surgical anatomy is depicted in fig. 11, and the appearance of the specimen (the plaque) and the repaired artery is shown in fig. 12.

Instead I patch it. Diane hands me a quarter-inch-wide strip of Dacron cloth, which I trim into an elongated, almond-shaped patch. Using fine nylon suture, I carefully sew the Dacron patch to the edges of the arterial incision, the carotid is closed.

We are ready now, to remove the latex ribbons from the internal and external carotid arteries. The back bleeding from these vessels will force the air, tiny bubbles, through the suture holes in the Dacron patch, so that when the clamp on the common carotid artery is removed, the reestablished blood flow will not carry air bubbles to the brain. That would cause a stroke.

I place a small gauze pad over the repaired artery. I press lightly on the Dacron patch and hold it firmly in place as I open the vascular clamp on the common carotid artery. Blood flow is reestablished to the right side of Mr. Crowe's brain. As expected, there is bleeding from the suture holes, but with finger pressure for a minute or two, the bleeding stops. The internal carotid artery, now patched and free of plaque, is pulsating nicely. (See figs. 11, 12.)

We irrigate the entire wound with saline, dry it with gauze pads and make sure that there is no bleeding in the wound. No bleeding at all. I peek at the clock. It is 11:15 A.M., 2 hours and 35 minutes into the surgery. We begin to close. I straighten out Mr. Crowe's head to take the tension off the wound. I remove the retractors. Then I sew the platysma muscle back together with a running stitch. I close the subcutaneous tissue with simple, absorbable sutures.

Dr. Randall, aware that we're almost finished, begins to wake him up. We close the skin with surgical staples, and cut a small strip of no-stick gauze, place it over the suture line, and hold it there with transparent tape. Then we wait. We wait to see if Mr. Crowe will wake up neurologically intact.

Rarely, in about 2 percent of cases, even when the procedure goes perfectly smoothly, some unnoticed air bubble or tiny piece of plaque can travel to the brain undetected in the reestablished blood flow and cause a stroke.

As we wait, I ask the student what the first sign of a stroke would be. He hesitates. I answer the question for him. "The first sign of a stroke is delayed arousal from anesthesia. Then when the patient does wake up, any sign of a stroke would appear on the opposite side of the body. We worked on the right, so a stroke would manifest itself as an inability to move his left arm, or left leg, or both, or an inability to speak."

First-year medical students know that the right side of the brain controls the left side of the body, and vice versa, but this student was really green. In another four or five years, when he has finished medical school and emerged from the cocoon of residency, he'll have changed into a confident, well-trained pediatrician. We forget we were once just as green. In the meantime, we'll continue to complain about the house staff. That's what surgeons do.

"Carotid artery surgery," I tell him, "is an operation which demands precision and experience. Any surgeon can inadvertently cause a stroke, but sloppy ones and beginners do it more often." Since the operation became popular in the late '60s, thousands of patients have been spared strokes, and a lot of surgeons have gotten ulcers while waiting, like we are now, for their patients to wake up. Usually, if a stroke does occur, you see it right away, on the operating room table. That's because we don't take our carotid endarterectomy patients off the operating table to the recovery room until they're fully awake. If they do awaken from anesthesia with a stroke, we put them back to sleep immediately and reopen the neck to make sure there's no clot in the artery that we've just cleaned out.

Mr. Crowe began to gag on the endotracheal tube. "Finally," I said. "He's starting to wake up."

"Look, he's moving his right arm," says the resident.

"That's nice," I tell him, "but it's the left side of his body we need to worry about."

"Look. He's moving his right leg," the student says.

"Great ... ask him to move his left arm."

Mr. Crowe's eyes remain shut. He's breathing nicely, and, according to the oxygen monitor, his blood oxygen levels are good. Dr. Randall removes the endotracheal tube. Mr. Crowe coughs. "Move your left arm. Wiggle your toes," she says, anxious to get him to the recovery room. Nothing. She lifts his left arm, and then lets it go. It flops back onto the O.R. table, flaccid.

"Stay sterile," I tell the student, "until we know he's neurologically intact." I'd been through this before, hundreds of times. It's nerve-wracking. Two or three more minutes go by. Then, Mr. Crowe, eyes still closed, slowly draws both knees up, and with his left hand, in slow motion, scratches his nose. "Okay," I say. "Take him to recovery." (See figs. 10, 11 for the anatomy of carotid artery surgery.)

Recovery room nurses are a tough lot. Our two recovery rooms each handle over twenty fresh post-ops at a time, all of whom have some degree of pain, nausea, or some other unpleasant bodily function going on. Each surgical condition has its own peculiar postoperative problems. Carotid endarterectomy patients like Mr. Crowe are subject to wide swings in their blood pressure.

The recovery room nurse's first job with each arriving patient is to record his vital signs: blood pressure, pulse rate, and temperature. In the case of the carotid endarterectomy patient, she also does a baseline neurological exam. The recovery room nurse checks the pupils. Are they equal? The face, is it symmetrical? Is the tongue pulled to one side? Do the toes wiggle? Is the hand grip equal on both sides? Can he talk?

In our hospital, carotid endarterectomy patients remain in the recovery room for four hours, then, if they are stable, they're transferred to a regular hospital room. About 2 percent of carotid endarterectomy patients suffer a stroke from the surgery. If a stroke does occur, it usually happens during the operation or within four hours post-op. Carotid artery stenting, which is still considered experimental, carries a stroke rate of about 11 percent, but in rare cases, where open surgery carries a prohibitive risk, it's still an option.

While the recovery room nurses were going over Mr. Crowe, the resident and I wrote postoperative orders. We checked Mr. Crowe's finger stick blood sugar, adjusted his insulin drip, and headed to the waiting area to reassure Betty. Then we went back to the O.R. for our next case, an open cholecystectomy.

Stroke in the Diabetic Patient

Stroke is a layman's term that describes a sudden loss of neurological function. The proper medical terminology is cerebrovascular accident (CVA). An ancient, no longer used term is apoplexy. All three words describe the same condition, partial loss of brain function due to loss of (oxygenated, arterial) blood supply to the sensitive brain cells. In diabetics, most strokes are caused by obstruction of an artery that supplies a particular part of the brain with blood. They're rarely caused by destruction of brain tissue from bleeding. Stroke is ranked as the third most frequent cause of death in the United States. It is also a leading cause of disability. Two million U.S. residents live isolated from society with brain damage, usually in the form of paralysis, due to strokes.

Diabetics are particularly prone to strokes because they tend to clog up their carotid arteries, the main blood supply to the brain, or to thrombose (clot-off) the smaller arteries within the brain. The diabetic's tendency toward high blood cholesterol and lipid levels and high blood pressure are responsible for the arterial blockages that result in strokes, heart attacks and peripheral vascular disease. The stroke rate in diabetics is almost three times that in non-diabetics. The use of cholesterol-lowering drugs, statins, along with proper diet and blood pressure control is an integral part of diabetic care. It is the primary means of preventing strokes.

Almost 80 percent of type 2 diabetics have high blood pressure. Correlate that statistic with the increased stroke rate and the conclusion is that high blood pressure is a major cause of stroke in the diabetic. The relationship between hypertension, diabetes and stroke has been studied extensively. It has been found that groups of diabetics who have been treated with blood pressure-lowering medication have 73 percent fewer strokes than do similar groups of diabetics who took no blood pressure-lowering medication.[1]

Mr. Crowe did not have a stroke. He had a warning sign, a transient ischemic attack (TIA). Lucky for him, because diabetics often have no warning — TIAs are more likely to precede strokes in non-diabetics than in diabetics.[2] He avoided a major stroke by surgical removal of his partially obstructing carotid artery plaque. He might have avoided surgery entirely, and he might never even have formed the atheromatous plaque if years earlier he had been placed on cholesterol-lowering and blood pressure-managing medications.

On the other hand, if Mr. Crowe had been a smoker, the entire process would have evolved years earlier. Cigarette smoking diabetics die decades earlier than non-smokers and are an endless source of work for the vascular surgeon.

Strokes are sudden and dramatic. They are more likely to occur in diabetics, and are deadlier in diabetics, but they represent only one of the neurological afflictions that are associated with poor diabetes control.

Chapter 10

DIABETES, IMPAIRED VISION, AND BLINDNESS

Blindness is one of those incapacitating conditions that hides its victims from society. Most blind people don't mingle. When you do encounter a blind person, he has likely been blind from an early age and has adjusted to the world about him. Those who lose their vision later in life have a tougher time. They are rarely seen, yet it is estimated that each year 24,000 people in the United States develop blindness as a complication of diabetes, and many more become severely visually impaired. In the U.S., diabetes is the leading cause of blindness in people between 20 and 74 years of age.[1]

In the diabetic, blindness and severe visual impairment are usually the result of a condition called *diabetic retinopathy*. Diabetic patients are subject to a higher incidence of cataracts and glaucoma, as well as dry eye.

In order to understand why diabetics are prone to visual impairment, a basic knowledge of eye anatomy is essential. Imagine the eye as a fluid-filled globe, a little smaller than a ping pong ball, with a hole in the front, the pupil, and a stem at the back, slightly off center, toward the ear — the optic nerve. Imagine that stem, that nerve, penetrating the globe and spreading out like a flower, say a buttercup, within it. The petals, tightly fused against the inner wall of the eye, represent the *retina*, the mirror-like surface upon which shines the beam of light passing through the pupil.

In the daytime, as the pupil contracts, the beam narrows. Like sunlight shining through a knothole in a barn wall, the bright spot of light hits a crucial area on the retina, a sequin-sized oval, the *macula*. At the center of the macula is a tiny crater, the *fovea*. The fovea, about the size of a poppy seed, contains only *cones*, the highly specialized photosensitive cells responsible for sharp color vision. There are no blood vessels in the fovea; if there were, they would block your vision.

This tiny target on the surface of the retina is responsible for just about all you see during daylight. At night, when the pupil dilates in order to let in more light, a larger part of the retina serves as a mirror on the world. But essentially the macula, which is no bigger than a hummingbird's eye, is the sole target of that light and provides your view of the world.

Diabetes attacks the retina — specifically its blood vessels. Diabetic eye damage is called *retinopathy*. Most often the extent of retinopathy is directly related to the number of years a person has had the disease. Studies have shown, for example, that when diabetes has been present for 16 years there is a 60 percent incidence of retinopathy.

The arteries and veins of the retina enter and leave the eye embedded within the optic nerve, the electric stem that connects the eyeball to the brain. The eye's blood vessels normally spread out over the retinal surface. Through the ophthalmoscope, they appear as through they've been painted on. The first sign of retinal damage by diabetes is the appearance of tiny, bead-like dilatations, called micro-aneurysms. The retinal vessels and micro-aneurysms are easily seen through an ophthalmoscope. Micro-aneurysms appear before symptoms occur; they are a sign of impending trouble.

Normal retinal blood vessels are lined with supporting cells called *pericytes*. As diabetes progresses, the pericytes disappear. This weakens the blood vessel walls. They begin to leak, first fluid, then blood. When leakage or bleeding occurs near the macula, swelling occurs. This is called macular edema or *maculopathy*. Left untreated, maculopathy is a major cause of blindness. As retinopathy progresses, the retinal blood vessels clot, close off, and scar down, depriving the retina of oxygen. The lack of oxygen stimulates the growth of numerous tiny new blood vessels, a process called neovascularization. Neovascularization is a healing process gone wrong. The flimsy new vessels often grow out of control. They may spread over the macula, block the light, cause loss of vision, leak plasma, bleed, or clot. As the clotted new vessels heal they form scars. As the scars contract, as all scars do, they may pull the retina from the inner surface of the eye, causing a sight-stealing retinal detachment. These pathologic events can occur in sequence or at random, dangerously near the macula or a safe distance from it. The damage can be observed directly through an ophthalmoscope, but arteriography, just as is used to examine the vessels of the heart or arteries of the legs, provides the best view.

People associate lasers with space age medicine, but lasers are rarely used except for cosmetic skin procedures and on the retina, where scalpels are of little use. (If a surgeon wants to use a laser on your hemorrhoids, beware. It's just a marketing device; find another doctor.) The most effective treatment for retinopathy is laser photocoagulation. (The word "laser" is an acronym coined from light amplification by stimulated emission of radiation.) The laser treatments stop leakage and bleeding and eliminate macular edema by obliterating the abnormal blood vessels. Up to 2,000 blasts of the laser may be needed to zap the spreading blood vessels and halt the damage. The normal blood vessels and the macula are carefully left intact, but if an errant blast of the laser hits the fovea, blindness occurs. Fortunately, this is very rare. Retinologists are good at what they do. The goal of the diabetic is to be aware that retinal damage can be present before it affects his vision. Retinopathy, like all diabetic complications, is progressive. Consequently, all diabetics should have a retinal examination at least once a year — even if they have no symptoms.

Pregnant diabetics are particularly prone to develop retinopathy. Because type 1 diabetes starts early in life, eye damage, retinopathy, may be present (but may be asymptomatic) prior to the pregnancy. The pregnant mother is at high risk for rapid progression of the problem. Pregnant women with pre-existing type 1 or 2 diabetes must be examined regularly throughout their pregnancy.

The type of retinal problem observed in type 1 diabetics may differ from that seen in type 2 diabetics. In type 1s, new blood vessel formation, neovascularization, is the predominant pathologic process. In type 2s, sudden, extensive capillary leakage is more common, and this explains why type 2 diabetics have a higher incidence of blinding macular edema. It is generally accepted that the presence of retinopathy (microvascular changes in the eye) signals the coexistence of diabetic nephropathy. The two diabetic complications frequently coexist.

The eyeball is filled with a clear, gel-like fluid called vitreous humor, which is 99 percent water. Occasionally, the diabetic with retinopathy, or with high blood pressure, can rupture a retinal vessel and bleed into this fluid. This can occur suddenly and severely impair vision. This out-of-the-blue event can occur by itself or be associated with a retinal tear. In this case, one treatment option is a complex surgical procedure involving removal of the vitreous humor, replacement with specialized saline solution, suture repair of the torn retina and laser photocoagulation, if needed.

The signature ocular complication of diabetes may be retinopathy,

Diabetes May Affect Any Part of the Eye, but Diabetic Retinopathy Is the Signature Pathology.

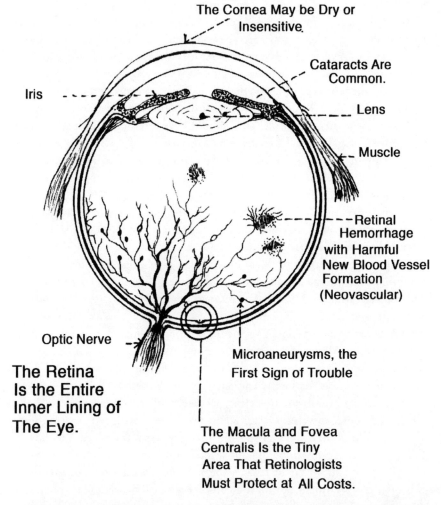

Fig. #14: The diabetic eye. Diabetes is a leading cause of blindness and visual impairment. Any part of the eye may be affected, but retinopathy is the signature pathology.

but the rest of the eye is affected as well. The sensitive corneal membrane may lose its sensitivity; the vitreous fluid that fills the eye may contract and pull the retina with it, detaching it; the iris may become inflamed, glaucoma may appear; and sudden elevations in blood sugar will change the osmolarity of body fluids and cause the lens to swell, which results in transient episodes of nearsightedness.[2] The complications of diabetes that affect the eye are not simple, and the procedures used to correct them are complex. There are ways, however, to minimize or even prevent retinopathy. Repeated studies have shown that careful control of one's blood sugar using the HbAlc as a guide, and keeping the blood pressure normal impedes the onset and progression of the condition.[3] Most important, because retinopathy is a silent, progressive condition and symptoms may not appear until the fovea is suddenly enveloped, regular retinal exams are vital (fig. 14).

Like all complications of diabetes retinopathy can be minimized by fastidious control of your blood sugar level — by keeping your HbAlc below 7. In fact, there appears to be a direct correlation between the risk of retinopathy and the HbAlc value. In 1997, The Expert Committee on the Diagnosis and Classification of Diabetes Mellitus determined that members of a very large study group, including the Pima Indians, whose blood glucose levels were below a certain level had little-to-no risk of retinopathy, but as individual's blood glucose levels rose, the prevalence of retinopathy followed in a linear fashion. In a more recent study of 28,000 individuals from nine countries it was determined that individuals with HbAlc values of less than 6.5 are at risk for type 2 diabetes. Indeed, this direct correlation between retinopathy as complication of diabetes, and HbAlc value underscores the usefulness of the HbAlc as a gauge of effective management as well as a diagnostic test. But keep in mind: in some cases retinopathy can develop quickly or even be the first sign of the disease. When retinopathy involves the macula, blindness is inevitable. So, the goal of the retinal surgeon is to protect the retina at all costs.[4]

Chapter 11

DIABETES, ORAL HEALTH, AND THE SURGEON

Diabetics have trouble with their teeth. Dental and periodontal (gum) disease are sometimes referred to as the sixth major complication of diabetes following heart disease, peripheral vascular disease, kidney disease, neuropathy and eye problems. The persistent high glucose levels that result from insulin resistance affect the periodontal tissues (the gums and bone around the teeth) causing inflammation or outright infection. Periodontal infections are extremely common in diabetics and correlate directly with their inability to keep their blood sugar in normal range.[1] Yet at the same time, severe periodontal disease causes high blood sugars. It's a self perpetuating cycle — high blood sugar leads to periodontal infection and periodontal infection leads to high blood sugars. Many surgeons fail to connect the ramifications of their diabetic patients severe gum disease to serious surgical complications. The obvious problem, well understood by anesthesiologists, is that during intubation (placement of a breathing tube), loose teeth are easily dislodged.

It is most important that patients inform their anesthesiologist if they have loose teeth. Not too long ago, I operated on a type 2 diabetic with an ulcerated leg. He had loose teeth from chronic gum disease. During the intubation, the anesthesiologist, who may have been a little rough, accidentally dislodged four of my patient's teeth. Using his laryngoscope and a long forceps he was able to fish three out of the patient's trachea. He was unaware that a fourth had tumbled further down into the patient's right bronchus, the main air channel to the right lung. The day after the surgery my patient spiked a high fever, developed chills, and began to cough. An X-ray exam showed a canine tooth in his chest; it showed aspiration pneumonia as well. A pulmonologist was called, and with my patient under sedation, he removed the tooth using a bronchoscope and wire basket. My patient recovered, but required a course of intravenous antibiotics to treat the pneumonia, and had an extended hospital stay.

Interestingly, there is a direct connection between chronic inflammation and infection from diabetic periodontal disease and the progression of peripheral vascular and coronary artery disease (heart attacks).[2] This may seem far-fetched to the layman (tooth and gum disease causing heart attacks), however, hard scientific evidence backs it up. The explanation is this: chronic inflammation anywhere in the body, be it from arthritis, lupus, or chronic gum disease, stimulates the release of inflammatory biomarkers into the bloodstream, These are measurable body chemicals which reflect your body's increased tendency towards excessive atherosclerosis and abnormal clotting, the ingredients for heart attack, stroke and peripheral artery disease.

Intensive oral (periodontal) care results in less chronic inflammation, which translates into fewer heart attacks, strokes and blocked arteries, fewer postoperative infections and better diabetic control. Currently, most dental health plans will cover two cleanings per year, but for the diabetic, more intensive oral care — say four cleanings per year — would result in a considerably lower incidence of periodontal pathology and save more teeth.[3] This would increase the financial burden on insurance companies and, by eliminating the need for more profitable dental care, it would decrease the dentist's income as well (which is not likely to happen in our medical market economy). The bottom line is — prevention beats treatment every time.

Periodontal infections are actually small abscesses between the teeth and the gum. They may contain hundreds of different types of bacteria. Some of these bacteria are extremely virulent. If they escape this small space between the gums and the teeth, the bacteria may travel through the bloodstream and implant in fresh surgical wounds, on heart valves, or around artificial joints and implanted devices like pacemakers. The result is severe infection and the need for major surgery and it happens more frequently than you might expect. Each time a diabetic patient bites an apple, brushes his teeth, or eats a meal, a struggle ensues between the bacteria launched into his bloodstream from his periodontal disease and his immune system.[4] I fear these circulating bacteria may settle in my patients' surgical wounds. This is reason enough for me to give prophylactic antibiotics to my surgical patients with detectable periodontal disease.

Dental caries, cavities, may be associated with poor diabetic control, but this has not been proven. Diabetics, to some degree, are chronically immunologically impaired; they can not fight infections as effectively as nondiabetics. For this reason they develop oral cavity conditions like candidiasis (fungal infections) and ulcerations of the mucosal lining of the mouth. Smoking and the use of dentures increases the severity of these conditions.

Dry mouth (xerostomia), loss of taste sensation, and a burning sensation of the tongue and mucous membranes are common manifestations of diabetic neuropathy. That the direct contact of sugar with the teeth causes cavities is no old wives' tale. It's verified by the observation that children with type 1 diabetes have fewer cavities. They're not allowed, for obvious reasons, to have sugary treats.

Periodontal disease, the sixth major complication of diabetes, and other chronic inflammatory conditions including obesity are not simply unwelcome byproducts of diabetes. Through their tendency to cause insulin resistance, they further elevate blood sugar levels and thus become risk factors for all the other diabetic complications.

Chapter 12

THE UNIQUE PROBLEM
OF TYPE 2 DIABETES
IN THE ELDERLY

Type 2 diabetes is appearing at an alarming rate in younger Americans, including the pediatric age group. We can trace this trend to lifestyle change and genetic factors. For the nation's elderly, it's a different story. The development of type 2 diabetes increases naturally with ageing, but making the diagnosis of diabetes can be difficult because the symptoms are not always typical. The classic initial symptoms in young and middle aged type 2s (and type 1s) are excessive thirst and appetite and frequent urination. Those usual symptoms can occur with elderly-onset diabetes, but they may be replaced or accompanied by episodes of confusion, incontinence, and dryness of the eyes and mouth. Adding to the confusion, even when their blood sugar levels are high, the elderly are less likely to spill sugar into their urine. As a result, many elderly-onset diabetics go undiagnosed. One study found that 6.9 percent of Americans, that's 2.4 million people, are unaware that they have the disease.[1] They attribute their symptoms to other causes. The usual methods of diagnosis (repeated fasting glucose levels) may miss 31 percent of new cases of diabetes in people over 65. For this reason, the diagnostic method of choice in the elderly is the more accurate two-hour glucose tolerance test.

Interestingly, the incidence of type 2 diabetes is site-specific. Where you live makes a difference.[2] For example, in Alaska, 13 percent of people over 65 have diabetes, whereas in Puerto Rico, 20 percent of the over 65 set are diabetic. In New York City, 12.5 percent of adults are diabetic.[3] One in every five hospital patients is diabetic, and here's a startling statistic: 25 percent of nursing home residents who are 65 or older are diabetic.[4] This is old data compiled by the National Nursing Home Survey of 2004; that number is undoubtedly higher now.

Elderly-onset type 2 diabetes poses challenges in diagnosis and treatment. The underlying mechanism is the same for people over 65 as it is with all type 2 diabetes — insulin resistance. The insulin produced by the pancreas is unable to act as a key to let glucose enter the cells for use as energy. Why the elderly develop insulin resistance is not entirely clear. Obesity does not appear to be a factor and the beta cells in the pancreas look normal.

The elderly diabetic may develop any of the usual complications, but is particularly prone to neuropathy. And that may compound an older individual's problems with balance and injury from falls. One form of motor neuropathy which is not often seen in younger diabetics is third cranial nerve palsy. When damaged by diabetic neuropathy, this nerve (also called the oculomotor nerve) causes double vision. Imagine a physician seeing a confused eighty-year-old who has suddenly lost bladder control and is seeing double. That doctor is not likely to place type 2 diabetes at the top of his list of possible diagnoses.

Memory impairment ranging from "senior moments" to Alzheimer's disease and depression is common in older people, but impaired brain function in elderly type 2 diabetics is specifically linked to these conditions. It is generally accepted that the diabetic's risk of developing Alzheimer's disease is 65–70 percent higher than the general population. Whether this is due to altered brain chemistry induced by elevated serum insulin levels or elevated blood glucose or an inability of brain cells to utilize insulin (insulin resistance) are hot research topics. It is interesting that postmortem microscopic examination of the brains of elderly diabetics show cellular changes that are similar to those found in Alzheimer's disease. Conversely, Alzheimer's patients, having diabetes-like microscopic brain pathology, have been referred to as having "diabetes of the brain." Older type 2 diabetics are particularly subject to defective working memory. But by keeping blood sugars in the normal range with proper medication and diet, cognitive impairment associated with type 2 diabetes can be minimized. Recent studies have shown that regular exercise, by stimulating blood flow to the brain, can slow the progression of Alzheimer's disease well.[5]

Elderly type 2 diabetics are prone to spontaneous drops in blood sugar. This may be manifested by sweating, nausea, and feeling faint. Adding to the problem, they may be more sensitive to insulin than their younger counterparts. This bollixed metabolic reaction to the usual doses of insulin also increases the risk of a sudden drop in blood sugar. With this in mind, some doctors feel that it may be wise to widen the acceptable range for glucose control in the elderly — for fastidious control is not worth the risk of precipitating a hypoglycemic attack.

Calcification of our blood vessel walls is part of our ageing process. As a vascular surgeon, I see and feel the blood vessels of many elderly people, diabetic and otherwise. There is a great variation in the appearance and "feel" of people's arteries. Some arteries are so soft and pliable that they are easily pinched closed between thumb and forefinger. Other arteries are so calcified and clogged that full force on a metal vascular clamp may break the clamp rather than pinch the artery closed. This observation, I admit, tempts me to believe that no medication could possibly benefit those patients with "lead pipe" arteries. Are these petrified people wasting their money on cholesterol-lowering drugs? The answer — surprise — is no! Calcification (arteriosclerosis) and plaque formation (atherosclerosis) are separate processes. Extensive collaborative studies involving thousands of patients have shown that the use of statin drugs (cholesterol, or plaque-lowering drugs) significantly reduces the heart attack rate (by 37 percent) in patients between the ages of 65 and 75. It's hard to argue with well-gathered statistics. The guidelines of the American Diabetes Association state that statin drugs should be used in all diabetics who are age forty or older.[6] One explanation, familiar to every vascular surgeon, is that arterial calcification is a segmental process. An artery may be hard as stone for an inch or two, then pliable as over-cooked pasta further along. Once started, a plaque in one segment of an artery tends to enlarge at a steady rate, whereas the clean, plaque-free segments of an artery (usually the part where there are no branches or pressure points), over time, tend to remain plaque-free.

Calcification occurs with ageing and is accelerated in diabetics, but calcification is not confined to blood vessels. Calcified fibroids hid the little fetus in Lydia Lang's uterus. Abdominal surgical scars often calcify like armor plates, and it's not unusual to see calcium in breast tumors where a typical pattern signifies malignancy. But there is one body structure that diabetics alone can calcify, and its presence, though just a curiosity, may flummox the uninformed physician. It's the vas deferens, that sperm-carrying tube that urologists cut when they do a vasectomy. The vas deferens runs from the testicle to the prostate, but, on its way, loops into the pelvis where, only when calcified, it can be seen on a simple abdominal X-ray film or a CAT scan.

Chapter 13

CATASTROPHE OR CURE

One can argue that the type 2 diabetes epidemic started when humans stopped eating to live and started living to eat, but it is more complicated than that. Those obese Zucker diabetic rats are intentionally created creatures. It took years of selective breeding and a forced lifestyle to make them diabetic. An analogy can be made between us, twenty-first century man, and those laboratory rats. The rats had no choice but to comply with their laboratory conditions. We, on the other hand, are capable of controlling at least some of the conditions in our "laboratory" — the diabetogenic-industrialized world. Nevertheless, our odds of becoming type 2 diabetics and suffering the complications have increased by over 70 percent in the last 15 years. We can control the rat's genetic makeup, but we have no control over our risk genes, at least for now. The risk genes we've always possessed plus the altered genes we inherit are coaxed into expression not by researchers, but through interaction with our diabetogenic environment.

Type 2 diabetes is the product of genetics and lifestyle, but lifestyle is imposed by the environment. Our environment and the lifestyle it demands can be changed only by making conscious decisions, knowledge-based decisions. The Zucker rats can't make decisions — but we can. The elimination of type 2 diabetes through sweeping societal and environmental changes is not likely, but by knowing the risks, biologic mechanisms, and probabilities, more individual inhabitants of our "laboratory" can avoid or minimize the disease. This has already been proven — it is possible to stop diabetes before it starts. Analysis of worldwide type 2 diabetes research indicates that lifestyle interventions reduce the number of new cases of type 2 diabetes by half, and proper use of blood pressure and cholesterol-lowering drugs by one third.[1]

We have the knowledge; we know why type 2 diabetes has become commonplace. Through "progress," we humans have created the perfect pathological niche. The Tohono/Pima Indians have shown us that our evolving socioeconomic status, our industrialized food supply, and the ever-decreasing need for personal energy expenditure are out of sync with our genetic makeup. At the same time, here, in the melting pot of the United States, through the natural intermixing of races (or of gene pools), the genetic requirements vital to the development of type 2 diabetes are becoming more prevalent. The spread of genes through inter-breeding of ethnic groups, *gene flow*, is partially responsible for increasing the appearance of type 2 diabetes throughout the world. We can't control our genetic makeup, but we can compensate by adjusting our lifestyles to keep our risk genes from expressing themselves.

In analyzing the outlook for diabetes as a worldwide problem, researchers and bio-statisticians throughout the globe hit the motherload when they determined that up to 70 percent of gestational diabetic women will themselves become permanent type 2 diabetics, and 50 percent of their offspring will become potential diabetics.[2] These impressive numbers are a product of our out-of-control, twenty-first century lifestyle. Many American women are overweight and have children late in life. The reality is, gestational diabetes disappears and may be forgotten with delivery of the baby. And the baby itself, having developed while in an altered metabolic milieu (exposed to high placental blood sugar while in the womb), is "imprinted" with a metabolism that increases its chances of becoming obese and diabetic later in life. In the final analysis, unchecked gestational diabetes translates into a self-perpetuating cycle of human suffering and healthcare expenditure.

Although obesity, eating habits, a sedentary lifestyle, and a variety of faulty genes are responsible for most cases of type 2 diabetes, scientists have uncovered many additional pathways to the problem. Type 2 diabetes of the elderly occurs in many previously healthy people who have only their longevity to blame. In this case it does not appear that the beta cells of the pancreas simply run out of steam; the problem is the gradual development of insulin resistance. Type 2 diabetes in the elderly is perhaps the one instance where we are stymied; science has yet to find a cause or means of prevention.

Obesity is the major risk factor for the onset of type 2 diabetes and, in view of the food culture we have created, the most difficult to eliminate. Social customs play a role. In Mauritania fat is beautiful; in India sweets are the symbol of prosperity, and in Spanish Harlem fast food restaurants are everywhere. Type 2 diabetes, however, is not always an eating disorder. Sometimes the genetic component is stronger than the lifestyle component.

According to the CDC, more than 60 percent of Americans are overweight and this segment of the population accounts for 80 percent of the type 2 diabetics. If the current trend continues, if we do not find a way to neutralize the effect of our post-industrial world on our genes and choices, within a few decades the world's population will be evenly divided between two types of people — diabetics and nondiabetics. We can wait for science to find a cure for society's ills, or, as educated individuals, we can do our best to avoid the disease in the first place.

Researchers working in rural India have shown that education, the institution of "population intervention programs," has succeeded in "reducing some of the risk factors responsible for type 2 diabetes and improving self management.[3]" Here in the U.S., researchers at Yale University studied over 170 overweight children and adolescents for twelve months. They recruited these nondiabetic children from their Pediatric Obesity Clinic. All had a BMI at or above the 95th percentile. With their parents' consent and the children's willingness to participate, these kids were divided into two groups: an "interventional" and a "control" group. The interventional (treated) group was exercised twice a week for fifty minutes, and dietitians, physicians, and nurse practitioners provided nutritional and activity counseling. The kids in the control group were seen in the Yale obesity clinic every six months. At the end of twelve months, the children in the treated group had significantly lowered their BMI and decreased their body fat by 9.2 kg compared to the control group. No surprise. But weight reduction was not the only benefit. Researchers took advantage of this experiment to measure the metabolic effect of weight reduction and exercise. By studying, in detail, blood insulin and glucose levels before and after each subject drank a flavored glucose drink, the researchers concluded, once again, that intensive lifestyle changes, by improving insulin sensitivity and lowering plasma insulin levels, can prevent or delay type 2 diabetes.[4]

Imagine if our schools were to educate all children. If school curricula, starting in the early grades, were designed to prevent diabetes and obesity by providing nutritional education courses and using appropriate lunch menus as a teaching tool. And if hospitals were to council potential diabetics rather than wait for them to develop the disease and profit from treating the complications. We need government-mandated reestablishment of physical education classes for children and fitness incentives for adults. We need prevention, not market-based facilitation. But, as it stands, true to the American way, we are dealing with the dual problems of obesity and type 2 diabetes by plugging them into our market economy. We, that is, our entrepreneurs, our healthcare system, our mass-produced food industry, our clothing companies, and our pharmaceutical concerns are facilitating obesity and type 2 diabetes and are cashing in on it. We produce wheelchairs that can barely fit through doorways, extra large clothing, scooters for knees that can no longer support the weight, weight-reduction operations, weight loss programs and all types of diet pills.

Two hundred and forty million diabetics are not going to change their lifestyles overnight. With this in mind, the global scientific community has been consumed with finding a cure, a magic bullet, a pill. But we are *Homo sapiens* — smart man. We, not the researchers or the healthcare establishment, must hold ourselves accountable for our health woes. Health conscious people need not understand all of the scientific intricacies in order to avoid or limit the disease, but they (we?) must be educated with regard to lifestyle risks.

Should the government get more involved? The answer, in a word, is yes. Our sometimes misguided sense of entitlement often overrides, even shuns, government authority. We know, for example, that smoking continues to be a major cause of illness and death. But if the government's campaign to curb cigarette smoking is a barometer of how we react to politicians meddling in our health decisions, then we can see that government-mandated warnings actually have made millions of people aware of the health hazards and given them the impetus to eliminate the risks of smoking.

Many Americans are oblivious to the tax burden foisted upon us by diabetes — 174 billion U.S. taxpayers' dollars in 2007 (according to the ADA). The average yearly cost of healthcare for each American diabetic is $13,242, compared to $2,560 for the non-diabetic.[5] The sheer cost is perhaps more of an incentive than the obesity/diabetes health crisis for long-overdue governmental oversight into our health-related eating decisions. Most Americans are nutritionally illiterate, and even smart people lack willpower. With that in mind, we must admit we need a watchdog, responsible central and local government, to regulate the food industry and encourage a healthy lifestyle. In 2009, the 111th United States Congress was to reintroduce both the Menu, Education and Labeling Act (MEAL Act), and the Labeling, Education and Nutrition Act (LEAN Act). The MEAL Act requires restaurant chains with twenty or more locations to post calorie, saturated fat, trans-fat and sodium contents on their menus and calorie counts next to each item on their menu boards. The LEAN Act would mandate that restaurant and grocery chains with twenty or more stores make nutritional data known to buyers before they reach the cash register. The Lean Act, if signed into law, would override all state and local regulations. The MEAL Act would serve as a national baseline, but allow local governments to add more health-promoting requirements. Medical organizations like the American Heart Association favor these moves, but the restaurants are opposed.[6] They argue that all restaurants should have the same requirements regardless of size. We would benefit, too, if more state governments, aside from California, strove to limit the number and type of fast food restaurants in a given area.

The United States Centers for Disease Control and Prevention Division of Diabetes Translation has studied the progression of diabetes. Based on its calculations, by the year 2050 the number of diabetics, primarily type 2s, will increase by an astounding 198 percent. The incidence of diabetes will increase 113 percent among Caucasians, 481 percent among Hispanics and 206 percent among African Americans. Other groups including Asians and Pacific Islanders will see a 158 percent rise in the incidence of diabetes.

Perhaps the most discouraging aspect of the Diabetes Report Card is this declaration by the Centers for Disease Control: "We also assume no advances in prevention, no possibility of a cure, no increases in life expectancy, no increases in screening or changes in diagnostic criteria."[7] This grave forecast portends an enormous burden on our health and our healthcare system and, unfortunately, assures that we vascular surgeons will have no shortage of work.

NOTES

The scientific information in this book comes from two sources, my personal experience as a surgeon and a review of the extensive, worldwide diabetes research, which I have translated into a readable format. There is no shortage of scientific information, for diabetes exists everywhere, and scientists, each with their special areas of interest, are desperate to find a cure. No doubt I have omitted some important facts, but my aim is to extract and splice together practical information that the layman can use to avoid type 2 diabetes or to minimize its complications.

Introduction

1. Ralph Waldo Emerson, *The Complete Writings of Ralph Waldo Emerson* (New York: William H. Wise & Co., 1929), 7.

2. Francis A. L'Esperance, Jr., and William A. James, Jr., *Diabetic Retinopathy, Clinical Evaluation and Management* (St. Louis: C.V. Mosby, 1981), 5, 197; N.S. Papaspyros, *The History of Diabetes Mellitus* 2nd ed. (Stuttgart: Georg Verlag, 1964), 7–9.

3. Sean Murphy, "Oklahoma City Mayor Puts City on a Diet," Associated Press, 3 January 2008; archived at www.msnbc.msn.com/id/22503467/.

Chapter 1

1. Christopher J. Schofield, Andrew D. Morris, M.D., et al., "Mortality and Hospitalization in Patients after Amputation, a Comparison between Patients with and without Diabetes," *Diabetes Care* (2006) 29:2252–2256.

2. George A Bender, *Great Moments in Medicine*, (Detroit: Northwood Institute Press, 1966), 48.

3. Suzanne Urverg Ratsimamanga, "Eugenia Jambolana: Madagascar," Malagasy Institute of Applied Research, retrieved from http://tcdc.undp.org/SIE/experiences/vol7/Eugenia%20Jambolana_Madagascar.pdf.

4. Spiros Fourlanos, M.D., Christine Perry, M.D., et al., "A Clinical Screening Tool Identifies Autoimmune Diabetes in Adults," *Diabetes Care* (May 2006) 29:970–975.

5. Thnamaija Tuomi, M.D., et al., "Improved Prandial Glucose Control with Lower Risk of Hypoglycemia with Nateglinide than with Glibenclamide in Patients with Maturity-Onset Diabetes of the Young Type 3," *Diabetes Care* (February 2006) 29:189–194.

6. MODY is the only type of diabetes for which specific genetic testing is available. See diabetesgenes.org, projects.exeter.ac.uk/diabetesgenes/mody/index.

7. http://en.wikipedia.org/wiki/Maturity_onset_diabetes_in_the_young.

8. Jesper Gromada, Isobel Franklin, and Claes B. Wollheim, "Alpha-cells of the Endocrine Pancreas: 35 Years of Research but the Enigma Remains," *Endocrine Reviews* 28 (1): 84–116.

9. Philip D. Hardt, Mathias D. Brendel, et al., "Is Pancreatic Diabetes (Type 3c Diabetes) Under Diagnosed and Mismanaged?" *Diabetes Care* (Supplement 2, February 2008) 31: s165–s169.

10. There is a genetic link between schizophrenia and type 2 diabetes. F. Gianfrancisco, R. White, et al., "Antipsychotic-Induced Type 2 Diabetes: Evidence from a Large Health Plan Data Base," *Journal of Clinical Pharmacology* (2003). 23: 328–335.

11. Stephanie De Wit, M.D., et al. "The Data Collection on Adverse Events of Anti-HIV Drugs (D:AD) Study," *Diabetes Care* (June 2008) 31: 1224–1229.

12. A.E. Krambeck, "Diabetes Mellitus and Hypertension Associated with Shock Wave Lithotripsy of Renal and Proximal Urethral Stones at 19 Years Follow-Up," *Journal of Urology* (1 May 2006) 175: 1742–1747.

13. Samuel Rahbar and origin of HbA1c: http://en.wikipedia.org/wiki/Samuel_Rahbar.

14. Catherine Buell, M.D., Dulcie Kermah, and Mayer B. Davidson, M.D., "Utility of A1C for Diabetes Screening in the 1999–2004 NHANES Population," *Diabetes Care* (September 2007) 30: 2233–2235.

15. Vinay Kumar, Ramzi S. Cotran, and Stanley L. Robbins, *Basic Pathology.* (Philadelphia: Saunders, 1992), 574.

16. Christophie De Block, M.D., et al. "Intensive Insulin Therapy in the Intensive Care Unit. Assessment by Continuous Glucose Monitoring," *Diabetes Care* (August 2006) 29: 1750–1756.

17. Pankaj Shah, Jeffrey Cui, Naifa L. Busaidy, Steven I. Sherman, and Victor R. Lavis, "Why is 'New' Hyperglycemia Dangerous in the Cancer Hospital?" (Abstract #1033-P), lecture presented at the American Diabetes Scientific Sessions, San Francisco, June 2008. Online at American Diabetes Association website; Diabetes PRO.

Chapter 2

1. The gene that predisposes to type 2 diabetes was discovered in research from de CODE Genetics, Reykjavik, Iceland, published Jan. 19, 2006 online by Medscape Medical News, Susan Jeffrey as first reported as a letter in the *J Nature Genetics* authored by Grant SFA, Thorleifson G., Reynisdottir L., Benediktsson R., Manolescu A., Sainz J., et. al.

2. Richard Beaser, M.D., and Amy P. Campbell, *The Joslin Guide to Diabetes* (New York: Simon & Schuster, 2005), 16.

3. Part of an excellent series on type 2 diabetes: N.R. Kleinfield, "Modern Ways Open India's Doors to Diabetes," *The New York Times,* 13 September 2006.

4. Catherine C. Cowie, et al., "Full Accounting of Diabetes and Pre–Diabetes in the U.S. Population in 1988–1994 and 2005–2006," *Diabetes Care* (February 2009) 32: 287–294.

5. "American Diabetes Association Clinical Practice Recommendations, 2005," *Diabetes Care* (2005, supplement 1) 28: s1–s79.

6. David M. Carroll, *The Year of the Turtle* (Charlotte, Vt.: Camden House, 1991).

7. Nathaniel Philbrick, *In the Heart of the Sea: The Tragedy of the Whaleship* Essex (New York: Penguin, 2000).

8. Andrew Skutch, *The Life of the Hummingbird* (New York: Vintage Books, 1973).

9. H. Klar Yaggi, M.D., Andre B. Araujo, and John B. McKinley, "Sleep Deprivation as a Risk Factor for Type 2 Diabetes," *Diabetes Care* (March 2006) 29: 657–661.

10. N.R. Kleinfield, "Living at an Epicenter of Diabetes, Defiance and Despair," *The New York Times*, 10 January 2006.

11. Padmini Balagopal, N. Kamalamma, Thackor G. Patel, M.D., and Ranjita Misra, "A Community-Based Diabetes Prevention and Management Education Program in a Rural Village in India," *Diabetes Care* (July 2008) 31: 1097–1104.

12. Carla McClain, "Southern Arizona, Epicenter of an Epidemic," *(Tucscon) Arizona Daily Star*, 18 July 2004.

13. Leslie O. Schulz, Peter H. Bennett, et al., "Effects of Traditional and Western

Environments on Prevalence of Type 2 Diabetes in Pima Indians in Mexico and the U.S.," *Diabetes Care* (August 2006) 29: 1866–1871.

14. Two similar scientific studies, which I have combined because they come to the same conclusion, prove that the environment plays a larger role in the development of type 2 diabetes than the number of risk genes you carry. The first study is James B. Meigs, M.D., et al., "Genotype Score in Addition to Common Risk Factors for Prediction of Type 2 Diabetes," *New England Journal of Medicine* (20 November 2008) 359: 2208–2219. The sister study is Valeriya Lyssenko, M.D., et al., "Clinical Risk Factors, DNA Variants, and the Development of Type 2 Diabetes," *New England Journal of Medicine* (20 November 2008) 359: 2220–2232.

15. Bruce Catton, *The American Heritage Short History of the Civil War* (New York: Dell Publishing, 1960).

Chapter 3

1. Henry S. Kahn, M.D., "The Lipid Accumulation Product Is Better than BMI for Identifying Diabetes, A Population Based Comparison," *Diabetes Care* (January 2006) 29: 151–153.

2. Susan B. Racette, Ellen M. Evans, Edward P. Weiss, et al., "Abdominal Adiposity Is a Stronger Predictor of Insulin Resistance than Fitness among 50 to 95 Year Olds," *Diabetes Care* (2006) 29: 673–678.

3. Iris Shai, Rui Jiang, M.D., et al., "Ethnicity, Obesity, and Risk of Type 2 Diabetes in Women, a Twenty Year Follow-Up Study," *Diabetes Care* (July 2006) 29: 1585–1590.

4. Susan Sam, M.D., Steven Haffner, M.D., Michael A. Davidson, M.D., Ralph B. Dagostino, Sr., M.D., Steven Feinstein, M.D., George Kondos, M.D., Alphonso Perez, M.D., Theodore Mazzone, M.D., "Relation of Abdominal Fat Deposits to Systemic Markers of Inflammation in Type 2 Diabetes," *Diabetes Care* (May 2009) 32: 932–937.

5. In healthy men and women, "moderate alcohol intake is associated with lower risk for type 2 diabetes." This is attributed to its positive effect on insulin, its lipid lowering effect and its "anti-inflammatory properties." Armin Inhof, M.D., Inez Plamper, M.S., Steffin Maier, M.S., Gerlinde Trischler, Wolfgang Koenig, M.D., "Effect of Drinking on Adiponectin in Healthy Men and Women," *Diabetes Care* (June 2003) 32: 1101–1103.

6. Debra Siefried Wind, "Type 2 Diabetes, Obesity and Bumblefoot: A Possible Correlation?" *Rat and Mouse Gazette*, June 2003, archived at www.rmca.org/Articles/ diabetestype2.htm.

7. Hidehiko Kondo, Ichiro Shimomura, Yoko Matsukawa, et al., "Association of Adiponectin Mutation with Type 2 Diabetes, a Candidate Gene for the Insulin Resistance Syndrome," *Diabetes* (2002) 51: 2325–2328.

8. Roger H. Unger, Yan Tang Zhou and Lelio Orci, "Regulation of Fatty Acid Homeostasis in Cells: Novel Role of Leptin," *Proceedings of the National Academy of Sciences* (2 March 1999) 96(5): 2327–2332.

9. Maarten E. Tushuizen, M.D., Mathis C. Bunk, M.D., et al., "Pancreatic Fat Content and B-Cell Function in Men with and without Type 2 Diabetes," *Diabetes Care* (November 2007) 30: 2916–2921.

10. Roger H. Unger, "Weapons of Lean Body Mass Destruction: The Role of Lipids in the Metabolic Syndrome," *Endocrinology* (2003) 144: 5159–5165.

11. "Do Bones Help Control Metabolism and Weight? Research Shows Skeleton to be Endocrine Organ, Crucial to Regulating Energy Metabolism; Osteocalcin Finding May Implicate Bone as Therapeutic Target for Type 2 Diabetes," Columbia University Medical Center press release, 9 August 2007, retrieved from www.cumc. columbia.edu/news/press_releases/karsenty _cell_osteocalcin_endocrine.html.

12. David M. Mutch, and Karine Clement, "Unraveling the Genetics of Human Obesity." PLoS Genetics, (29 December 2006) 2 (12):. e 188.

13. Vojtech Hainer, M.D., Herman Toplak, M.D., and Asimina Mitrakau, M.D., "Treatment Modalities of Obesity, What Fits Whom?" *Diabetes Care* (Supplement 2, February 2008) 31: s269–s277.

14. John Dixon, et al., "Adjustable Gastric Banding and Conventional Therapy for

Type 2 Diabetes," *Journal of the American Medical Association* (23 January 2008) 299: 316–323.

15. There is an "intestinal component" responsible for the disappearance of type 2 diabetes following weight loss surgery. Dr. Rubino provides the statistics that show the effectiveness of the various types of weight loss surgery in Francesco Rubino, M.D., "Is Type 2 Diabetes an Operable Intestinal Disease? A Provocative yet Reasonable Hypothesis," *Diabetes Care* (February 2008, supplement 2) 31: s290–s296.

16. A thorough discussion of the effectiveness and complications of bariatric surgery is presented by Guntram Schernithaner, M.D., and John M. Morton, M.D., "Bariatric Surgery in Patients with Morbid Obesity and Type 2 Diabetes," *Diabetes Care* (February 2008 supplement 2) 30: s297–s302.

17. Sharon LaFraniere, and Rukmini Callimachi, "In Mauritania, Seeking to End an Overfed Ideal," *The New York Times,* 4 July 2007.

18. Louis B. Sardinha, et al., "Objectively Measured Time Spent Sedentary Is Associated with Insulin Resistance Independent of Overall and Central Body Fat in 9- to 10-Year-Old Portuguese Children," *Diabetes Care* (March 2008) 31: 569–575.

19. Dana Dabelea, M.D., "The Predisposition to Obesity and Diabetes in Offspring of Diabetic Mothers," *Diabetes Care* (July 2007, supplement 2) 30: s169–s174.

20. Elizabeth J. Meyer-Davis, et al., "Breast-Feeding and Risk for Childhood Obesity," *Diabetes Care* (October 2006) 29: 2231–2237.

21. Maike C. Epins, Maria E. Craig, et al., "Prevalence of Diabetes Complications in Adolescents with Type 2 Compared with Type 1 Diabetes," *Diabetes Care* (June 2006) 29: 1300–1306.

22. H. Yokoyama, M. Okudaria, A. Sato, et al., "Higher Incidence of Diabetic Neuropathy in Type 2 than in Type 1 Diabetics in Early Onset Diabetes in Japan," *Kidney International* (2000) 58: 302–311.

23. Shelagh A. Mulvaney, et al., "Parent Perceptions for Adolescents with Type 2 Diabetes," *Diabetes Care* (May 2006) 29: 993–997.

Chapter 4

1. S.Y. Chu, W.M. Callaghan, M.D., et al., "Maternal Obesity and Risk of Gestational Diabetes Mellitus," *Diabetes Care* (2007) 30: 2070–2076.

2. Ibid.

3. Terrence T. Lao, M.D., Lai-Fong Ho, et al., "Maternal Age and Prevalence of Gestational Diabetes Mellitus," *Diabetes Care* (April 2006) 29: 948.

4. F.L. Gaudier, J.C. Hauth, et al., "Recurrence of Gestational Diabetes Mellitus," *Obstetrics and Gynecology* (1992) 80:755–780.

5. Assiamira Ferrara, M.D., "Increasing Prevalence of Gestational Diabetes Mellitus: A Public Health Perspective," *Diabetes Care* (July 2006, supplement) 30: s141–s146.

6. Catherine Kim, M.D., Laura N. McEwen, John D. Piette, et al., "Risk Perception for Diabetes among Women with Histories of Diabetes Mellitus," *Diabetes Care* (September 2007) 30: 2281–2286.

7. Dana Dabelea, M.D., "The Predisposition to Obesity and Diabetes in Offspring of Diabetic Mothers," *Diabetes Care* (July 2007, supplement 2) 30: s169–s174.

8. Robert G. Moses, M.D., Megan Barker, A.P.D., Meagen Winter, A.P.D., Peter Petocz, Ph.D., Jennie C. Brand-Miller, Ph.D., "Can a Low-Glycemic Index Diet Reduce the Need for Insulin in Gestational Diabetes Mellitus?" *Diabetes Care* (June 19, 2009) 32: 996–1000.

9. Cuilin Zhang, M.D., Simin Liu, M.D., Caren G. Solomon, M.D., and Frank B. Hu, M.D., "Dietary Fiber Intake, Dietary Glycemic Load, and the Risk for Diabetes Mellitus," *Diabetes Care* (October 2006) 29: 2223–2230.

10. Diane M. Reader, "Medical Nutrition Therapy and Life Style Interventions," *Diabetes Care* (July 2007, supplement 2) 30: s188–s193.

11. Danielle Symons Downs and Jan S. Ulbrecht, M.D., "Understanding Exercise Beliefs and Behaviors in Women with Gestational Diabetes Mellitus," *Diabetes Care* (February 2006) 29: 236–240.

12. Robert Ratner, M.D., "Prevention of Type 2 Diabetes in Women with Previous Gestational Diabetes," *Diabetes Care* (July 2007, supplement 2) 30: s242–s245.

Chapter 5

1. Vinay Kumar, Ramzi S. Cotran and Stanley L. Robbins, *Basic Pathology* (Philadelphia: Saunders, 1992), 579.
2. Lea Sorensen, Linda Molyneaux and Dennis K. Yue, "The Relationship among Pain, Sensory Loss, and Small Nerve Fibers in Diabetes," *Diabetes Care* (April 2006) 29: 883–887.
3. A. Gordon Smith, M.D., et al., "Life Style Intervention for Pre–Diabetic Neuropathy," *Diabetes Care* (June 2006) 29: 1204–1299.
4. Zachary T. Bloomgarden, M.D., "Diabetic Neuropathy," *Diabetes Care* (March 2008) 38: 620.
5. Urinary incontinence is a common — perhaps the most common — complication in obese, diabetic obese women, but African American, Asian and non-white Hispanic diabetic women are no more likely to experience this problem than non-diabetic women. Suzanne Phelan et al., "Prevalence and Risk Factors for Urinary Incontinence in Overweight and Obese Diabetic Women," *Diabetes Care* (August 2009) 32: 1391–1397.
6. V.A. Shepherd, "Bioelectricity and the Rhythms of Sensitive Plants: The Biophysical Research of Jagadis Chandra Bose," *Current Science Online,* www.ias.ac.in/currsci/jul10/articles33.htm.

Chapter 6

1. Igor E. Kostantinov, M.D., Nicolai Mejevoi, M.D., Nicolai M. Anichkov, M.D., et al., "Nikolai N. Anichkov and His Theory of Atherosclerosis," *Journal of the. Texas Heart Institute* 33 (November 2006): 417–423.
2. Throughout the world, and especially in India where people in rural areas often go shoeless, diabetic foot problems abound and are the most common reason for hospitalization of the diabetic. John M. Giurini, "Diabetic Foot Management" (educational course, Department of Surgery, Beth Israel Deaconess Medical Center and the Joslin Diabetes Center, Nov. 9–10, 2000).
3. Edouard Ghanassia, M.D., Laettia Villon, M.D., et al., "Long Term Outcome and Disability of Diabetic Patients Hospitalized for Diabetic Foot Ulcers," *Diabetes Care* (July 2008) 31:1288–1292.
4. Jo C. Dumville, Gill Worthy, J. Martin Bland, Nicky Cullum, Christopher Dowson, Cynthia Iglesias, Joanne L. Mitchell, E. Andrea Nelson, Marta O. Soares, David J. Torgerson, "Larval Therapy for Leg Ulcers (VenUS II): Randomized Controlled Trial on Behalf of the VenUS II Team," *British Medical Journal* (March 25, 2009) 338: b773.
5. John M. Giurini, "Diabetic Foot Management" (educational course, Department of Surgery, Beth Israel Deaconess Medical Center and the Joslin Diabetes Center, Nov. 9–10, 2000).
6. Kimball C. Atwood IV, M.D., Elizabeth Woeckner, Robert S. Baratz, M.D. and Wallace A. Sampson, M.D., "Why the NIH Trial to Assess Chelation Therapy (TACT) Should Be Abandoned," *The Medscape Journal of Medicine* 2008) 10(5): 115. Retrieved from http://www.pubmedcentral.nih.gov/articlerender.fcgi?artid=2438277.
7. The problem of unexploded land mines: http://www.unicef.org/graca/mines.htm.
8. David J. Margolis, M.D., Ole Hofstad, and Harold I. Feldman, M.D., "The Association between Renal Failure and Foot Ulcer or Lower Extremity Amputation in Patients with Diabetes," *Diabetes Care* (July 2008) 31: 1331–1336; American Diabetes Association statistic cited in *Diabetes Care* (2003) 26:3333–3341.
9. Guiseppe Lepore, M.D., Maria Maglio, M.D., Carlo Cuni, M.D., et al., "Poor Glucose Control in the Year before Admission as a Powerful Predictor of Amputation in Hospitalized Patients with Foot Ulceration," *Diabetes Care* (August 2006) 29: 1985.
10. Laura M. McEwen, William H. Herman, M.D., et al., "Diabetes Reporting as a Cause of Death, Results from the Translating Results into Action for Diabetes (TRIAD) Study," *Diabetes Care* (February 2006) 29: 247–253.

Chapter 7

1. Frans J. Th. Wackers, M.D., et al., "Resolution of Asymptomatic Myocardial

Ischemia in Patients with Type 2 Diabetes in the Detection of Ischemia in Asymptomatic Diabetics (DIAD) Study," *Diabetes Care* (November 2007) 30: 2892–2898.

2. A. P. Kengne, G.B. Amoah, and J.C. Mbanya, "Cardiovascular Complications of Diabetes Mellitus in Sub-Saharan Africa," *Circulation* (2005) 112: 3592–3601.

3. The American Diabetes Association recommends that all diabetics over 40 take statin medication, *Diabetes Care* (2006, supplement 1) 29:s4–s42.

4. American Heart Association statistic.

5. Shelly E. Ellis, Tom A. Elasy, et al., "Exercise and Glycemic Control in Diabetes," *Journal of the American Medical Association* (2001) 286: 2941–2942; and Normand G. Boulé, Elizabeth Haddad, M.D., et al., "Effects of Exercise on Glycemic Control and Body Mass in Type 2 Diabetes Mellitus; A Meta-analysis of Controlled Clinical Trials," *Journal of the American Medical Association* (2001) 286: 1218–1227.

6. Michael Ho, M.D., E.D. Peterson., L. Wang, et al., "Incidence of Death and Acute Myocardial Infarction Associated with Stopping Clopidogrel after Acute Coronary Syndrome." *Journal of the American Medical Association* (2008) 99(5): 532–539.

7. I.M. Stratton, et al., "Association of Glycemia with Macrovascular and Microvascular Complications of Type 2 Diabetes (UKPDS 35): Prospective Observational Study," *British Medical Journal* (2000) 321: 405–412.

8. Jay S. Skyler, M.D., et al., "Intensive Glycemic Control and the Prevention of Cardiovascular Events: Implications of the ACCORD, ADVANCE, and VA Diabetes Trials," *Diabetes Care* (2009) 32:187–192.

Chapter 8

1. Vinay Kumar, Ramzi S. Cotran, and Stanley L. Robbins, *Basic Pathology* (Philadelphia: Saunders, 1992), 576.

2. Takeisi Oomichi, M.D., Masonori Emoto, M.D., et al., "Impact of Glycemic Control on Survival of Diabetic Patients on Chronic Regular Hemodialysis, a 7-year Observational Study," *Diabetes Care* (July 2006) 29: 1496–1500.

3. Jay L. Xue, Jennie Z. Ma, Thomas A. Lewis, and Allan J. Collins, "Forecast of the Number of Dialysis Patients in the United States to the Year 2010," *Journal of the American Society of Nephrology* (2001) 12: 2753–2758.

4. American Diabetes Foundation statistic.

5. History of hemodialysis: http://www.fmc-ag.com/internet/fmc/fmcag/neu/fmc pub.nsf/Content/Dialysis_Compact_2004_0.

6. Richard Perez-Pena, "As Increase in Diabetes Destroys More Kidneys, New York Dialysis Lags," *The New York Times*, 28 December 2006.

7. An on-target description of the dialysis business and the tough life of dialysis patients: Andrew Pollack, "The Dialysis Business: Fair Treatment?" *The New York Times*, 16 September 2007.

8. Ibid.

Chapter 9

1. J. Tuomilehto, et al., "Effects of Calcium-Channel Blockade in Older Patients with Diabetes and Systolic Hypertension," *New England Journal of Medicine* (1999) 340: 677–684.

2. Ellen L. Air, M.D., and Brett M. Kissela, "Diabetes, the Metabolic Syndrome, and Ischemic Stroke, Epidemiology and Possible Mechanisms," *Diabetes Care* (December 2007) 30: 3131–3140.

Chapter 10

1. Philip M. Clarke, Judit Simon, M.D., Carol A. Cull, and Rudy R. Holman, "Assessing the Impact of Visual Acuity on Quality of Life in Individuals with Type 2 Diabetes Using the Short Form-36," *Diabetes Care* (July 2006) 29: 1506–1511.

2. Duane, Thomas David, William Tasnan, M.D., and Edward A. Jaeger, *Duane's Clinical Ophthalmology* (Philadelphia: Lippincott-Raven, revised edition, 1996).

3. Francis A. L'Esperance and William A. James Jr., *Diabetic Retinopathy, Clinical Evaluation and Management* (St. Louis: C.V. Mosby, 1981) 121.

4. The direct relationship between retinopathy and the HbA1c helps establish the HbA1c as a diagnostic test: The International Expert Committee (David M. Nathan, corresponding author), "International Expert Committee Report on the Role of the A1C Assay in the Diagnoses of Diabetes," *Diabetes Care* 32:1327–1334, July 2009.

Chapter 11

1. Jonathan A. Ship, "Diabetes and Oral Health: An Overview," *Journal of the American Dental Association* (4 April 2003) 134: 4S–10S.
2. Maurizio S. Tonetti, et al., "Treatment of Periodontitis and Endothelial Function," *The New England Journal of Medicine* (1 March 2007) 356: 911–920.
3. Personal communication with dental plan administrator who does not wish to be named.
4. Marie E. Ryan, Oana Carnu, and Ruth Tenzler. "The Impact of Periodontitis on Metabolic Control and Risk for Diabetic Complications." *RDH Magazine*, 19 July 2007, archived at www.rdhmag.com/display_article/300572/108/none/none/Oart/THE-IMPACT-OF-PERIODONTITIS-ON-METABOLIC-CONTROL-AND-RISK-FOR-DIABETIC-COMPLICTION.

Chapter 12

1. Elizabeth Selven, Josef Coresh, M.D., and Frederick L. Brancati, M.D., "The Burden and Treatment of Diabetes in Elderly Individuals in the U.S.," *Diabetes Care* (November 2006) 29: 2415–2419.
2. Diabetes data and trends from the U.S. Centers for Disease Control and Prevention: http://apps.nccd.cdc.gov/ddtstrs/.
3. Lorna E. Thorpe, et al., "Prevalence and Control of Diabetes and Impaired Fasting Glucose in New York City," *Diabetes Care* (January 2009) 32: 57–62.
4. Helane E. Resnick, Janice Heineman, Robin Stone, et al., "Diabetes in U.S. Nursing Homes, 2004," *Diabetes Care* (February 2008) 31: 287–288.
5. Christopher M. Ryan, et al. "Improv-

ing Metabolic Control Leads to Better Working Memory in Adults with Type 2 Diabetes," *Diabetes Care* (February 2006) 20: 345–351; and Medha Munshi, M.D., et al., "Cognitive Dysfunction Is Associated with Poor Diabetes Control in Older Adults," *Diabetes Care* (August 2006) 29: 1794–1700.
6. H. Andrew W. Neil, et al., "Collaborative Atrovastatin Diabetes Study (CARDS), Analysis of Efficacy and Safety in Patients Aged 65–75 Years at Randomization," *Diabetes Care* (November 2006) 29: 2378–2384.

Chapter 13

1. Zachary T. Bloomgarden, M.D., "Approaches to Treatment of Pre–Diabetes and Obesity and Promising New Approaches to Type 2 Diabetes," *Diabetes Care* 31 (July 2008): 1461–1466.
2. Teresa A. Hillier, M.D., Kathryn L. Pedula, Mark M. Schmidt, et al., "Childhood Obesity and Metabolic Imprinting: The Ongoing Effect of Maternal Hyperglycemia," *Diabetes Care* (September 2007) 30: 2287–2292.
3. Padmini Balagopal, N. Kamalamma, Thackor G. Patel, M.D., and Ranjita Misra, "A Community-Based Diabetes Prevention and Management Education Program in a Rural Village in India," *Diabetes Care* (July 2008) 31: 1097–1104.
4. Milissa Shaw, Mary Savoye, Anna Calle, M.D., et al., "Effect of a Successful Lifestyle Program on Insulin Sensitivity and Glucose Tolerance in Obese Youth," *Diabetes Care* (January 2009) 32: 45–47.
5. Peter Gaede, M.D., et al., "Cost-Effectiveness of Intensified Versus Conventional Multifactorial Intervention in Type 2 Diabetes (Results and Projections from the Steno-2 Study)," *Diabetes Care* (August 2008) 31: 1510–1515.
6. Paul Frumkin, "Industry Watchdogs Prepare to Battle over Dueling Menu-Labeling Mandates," *Nations Restaurant News*, December 2008.
7. K.M. Venkat Narayan, M.D., et al., "Impact of Recent Increase on Future Diabetes Burden, U.S. 2005–2050," *Diabetes Care* (September 2006) 29: 2114–6.

BIBLIOGRAPHY

Air, Ellen L., M.D., and Brett M. Kissela. "Diabetes, the Metabolic Syndrome, and Ischemic Stroke, Epidemiology and Possible Mechanisms," *Diabetes Care* (December 2007) 30: 3131–3140.

Atwood, Kimball C. IV, M.D., Elizabeth Woeckner, Robert S. Baratz, M.D., and Wallace A. Sampson, M.D. "Why the NIH Trial to Assess Chelation Therapy (TACT) Should Be Abandoned." *The Medscape Journal of Medicine* (2008) 10(5): 115. Retrieved from http://www.pubmedcentral.nih.gov/articlerender.fcgi?artid=2438277.

Balagopal, Padmini, N. Kamalamma, Thackor G. Patel, M.D., and Ranjita Misra. "A Community-Based Diabetes Prevention and Management Education Program in a Rural Village in India." *Diabetes Care* (July 2008) 31: 1097–1104.

Beaser, Richard, M.D., and Amy P. Campbell. *The Joslin Guide to Diabetes.* New York: Simon & Schuster, 2005.

Bender, George A. *Great Moments in Medicine*, Detroit: Northwood Institute Press, 1966.

Bloomgarden, Zachary T., M.D. "Approaches to Treatment of Pre-Diabetes and Obesity and Promising New Approaches to Type 2 Diabetes." *Diabetes Care* 31 (July 2008): 1461–1466.

———. "Diabetic Neuropathy." *Diabetes Care* (March 2008) 38: 620.

Boulé, Normand G., Elizabeth Haddad, M.D., et al. "Effects of Exercise on Glycemic Control and Body Mass in Type 2 Diabetes Mellitus; A Meta-analysis of Controlled Clinical Trials." *Journal of the American Medical Association* (2001) 286: 1218–1227.

Buell, Catherine, M.D., Dulcie Kermah, and Mayer B. Davidson, M.D. "Utility of A1C for Diabetes Screening in the 1999–2004 NHANES Population." *Diabetes Care* (September 2007) 30: 2233–2235.

Callimachi, Rukmini, and Sharon La Franiere. "In Mauritania, Seeking to End an Overfed Ideal. *The New York Times,* 4 July 2007.

Carroll, David M. *The Year of the Turtle.* Charlotte, Vt.: Camden House, 1991.

Catton, Bruce. *The American Heritage Short History of the Civil War.* New York: Dell Publishing, 1960.

Chu, S.Y., W.M. Callaghan, M.D., et al. "Maternal Obesity and Risk of Gestational Diabetes Mellitus." *Diabetes Care* (2007) 30: 2070–2076.

Clarke, Philip M., Judit Simon, M.D., Carol A. Cull, and Rudy R. Holman. "Assessing the Impact of Visual Acuity on Quality of Life in Individuals with Type 2 Diabetes Using the Short Form-36." *Diabetes Care* (July 2006) 29: 1506–1511.

Cowie, Catherine C., et al. "Full Accounting of Diabetes and Pre-Diabetes in the U.S. Population in 1988–1994 and 2005–2006." *Diabetes Care* (February 2009) 32: 287–294.

Dabelea, Dana, M.D. "The Predisposition to Obesity and Diabetes in Offspring of Diabetic Mothers." *Diabetes Care* (July 2007, supplement 2) 30: s169–s174.

De Block, Christophie, M.D., et al. "Intensive Insulin Therapy in the Intensive Care Unit. Assessment by Continuous Glucose Monitoring." *Diabetes Care* (August 2006) 29: 1750–1756.

De Wit, Stephanie, M.D., et al. "The Data Collection on Adverse Events of Anti-HIV Drugs (D:AD) Study." *Diabetes Care* (June 2008) 31: 1224–1229.

Dixon, John, et al. "Adjustable Gastric Banding and Conventional Therapy for Type 2 Diabetes." *Journal of the American Medical Association* (23 January 2008) 299: 316–323.

"Do Bones Help Control Metabolism and Weight? Research Shows Skeleton to be Endocrine Organ, Crucial to Regulating Energy Metabolism; Osteocalcin Finding May Implicate Bone as Therapeutic Target for Type 2 Diabetes." Columbia University Medical Center press release, 9 August 2007. Retrieved from www. cumc.columbia.edu/news/press_ releases/karsenty_cell_osteocalcin_endoc rine.html.

Downs, Danielle Symons, and Jan S. Ulbrecht, M.D. "Understanding Exercise Beliefs and Behaviors in Women with Gestational Diabetes Mellitus." *Diabetes Care* (February 2006) 29: 236–240.

Duane, Thomas David, William Tasnan, M.D., and Edward A. Jaeger. *Duane's Clinical Ophthalmology.* Philadelphia: Lippincott-Raven, revised edition, 1996.

Dumville, Jo C., Gill Worthy, J. Martin Bland, Nicky Cullum, Christopher Dowson, Cynthia Iglesias, Joanne L. Mitchell, E. Andrea Nelson, Marta O. Soares, David J. Torgerson. "Larval Therapy for Leg Ulcers (VenUS II): Randomized Controlled Trial on Behalf of the VenUS II Team." *British Medical Journal* (March 25, 2009) 338: b773.

Ellis, Shelly E., Tom A. Elasy, et al. "Exercise and Glycemic Control in Diabetes." *Journal of the American Medical Association* (2001) 286: 2941–2942.

Epins, Maike C., Maria E. Craig, et al. "Prevalence of Diabetes Complications in Adolescents with Type 2 Compared with Type 1 Diabetes." *Diabetes Care* (June 2006) 29: 1300–1306.

Ferrara, Assimira, M.D. "Increasing Prevalence of Gestational Diabetes Mellitus: A Public Health Perspective." *Diabetes Care* (July 2006, supplement) 30: s141–s146.

Fourlanos, Spiros, M.D., et al. "A Clinical Screening Tool Identifies Autoimmune Diabetes in Adults." *Diabetes Care* (May 2006) 29: 970–975.

Frumkin, Paul. "Industry Watchdogs Prepare to Battle over Dueling Menu-Labeling Mandates." *Nations Restaurant News*, December 2008.

Gaede, Peter, M.D., et al. "Cost-Effectiveness of Intensified Versus Conventional Multifactorial Intervention in Type 2 Diabetes (Results and Projections from the Steno-2 Study)." *Diabetes Care* (August 2008) 31: 1510–1515.

Gaudier, F.L., J.C. Hauth, et al. "Recurrence of Gestational Diabetes Mellitus." *Obstetrics and Gynecology* (1992) 80:755–780.

Ghanassia, Edouard, M.D., Laettia Villon, M.D., et al. "Long Term Outcome and Disability of Diabetic Patients Hospitalized for Diabetic Foot Ulcers." *Diabetes Care* (July 2008) 31:1288–1292.

Giurini, John M. "Diabetic Foot Management." (Educational course, Department of Surgery, Beth Israel Deaconess Medical Center and the Joslin Diabetes Center, Nov. 9–10, 2000).

Gromada, Jesper, Isobel Franklin, and Claes B. Wollheim. "Alpha-cells of the Endocrine Pancreas: 35 Years of Research but the Enigma Remains." *Endocrine Reviews* 28 (1): 84–116.

Hainer, Vojtech, M.D., Herman Toplak, M.D., and Asimina Mitrakau, M.D. "Treatment Modalities of Obesity, What Fits Whom?" *Diabetes Care* (Supplement 2, February 2008) 31: s269–s277.

Hardt, Philip D., Mathias D. Brendel, et al. "Is Pancreatic Diabetes (Type 3c Diabetes) Under Diagnosed and Mismanaged?" *Diabetes Care* (Supplement 2, February 2008) 31: s165–s169.

Hillier, Teresa A., M.D., Kathryn L. Pedula, Mark M. Schmidt, et al. "Childhood Obesity and Metabolic Imprinting: The Ongoing Effect of Maternal Hyperglycemia." *Diabetes Care* (September 2007) 30: 2287–2292.

Ho, Michael, M.D., E.D. Peterson., L. Wang, et al. "Incidence of Death and Acute Myocardial Infarction Associated with Stopping Clopidogrel after Acute

Coronary Syndrome." *Journal of the American Medical Association* (2008) 99(5): 532–539.

Inhof, Armin, M.D., Inez Plamper, M.S., Steffin Maier, M.S., Gerlinde Trischler, Wolfgang Koenig, M.D. "Effect of Drinking on Adiponectin in Healthy Men and Women." *Diabetes Care* (June 2003) 32: 1101–1103.

Kahn, Henry S., M.D. "The Lipid Accumulation Product Is Better than BMI for Identifying Diabetes, A Population Based Comparison." *Diabetes Care* (January 2006) 29: 151–153.

Kengne, A.P., G.B. Amoah, and J.C. Mbanya. "Cardiovascular Complications of Diabetes Mellitus in Sub-Saharan Africa." *Circulation* (2005) 112: 3592–3601.

Kim, Catherine, M.D., Laura N. McEwen, John D. Piette, et al. "Risk Perception for Diabetes among Women with Histories of Diabetes Mellitus." *Diabetes Care* (September 2007) 30: 2281–2286.

Kleinfield, N.R. "Living at an Epicenter of Diabetes, Defiance and Despair." *The New York Times*, 10 January 2006.

_____. "Modern Ways Open India's Doors to Diabetes." *The New York Times*, 13 September 2006.

Kondo, Hidehiko, Ichiro Shimomura, Yoko Matsukawa, et al. "Association of Adiponectin Mutation with Type 2 Diabetes, a Candidate Gene for the Insulin Resistance Syndrome." *Diabetes* (2002) 51: 2325–2328.

Kostantinov, Igor E., M.D., Nicolai Mejevoi, M.D., Nicolai M. Anichkov, M.D., et al. "Nikolai N. Anichkov and His Theory of Atherosclerosis." *Journal of the Texas Heart Institute* 33 (November 2006): 417–423.

Kumar, Vinay, Ramzi S. Cotran, and Stanley L. Robbins. *Basic Pathology.* Philadelphia: Saunders, 1992.

Lao, Terrence T., M.D., Lai-Fong Ho, et al. "Maternal Age and Prevalence of Gestational Diabetes Mellitus." *Diabetes Care* (April 2006) 29: 948.

L'Esperance, Francis A., Jr., and William A. James Jr. *Diabetic Retinopathy, Clinical Evaluation and Management.* St. Louis: C.V. Mosby, 1981.

Lepore, Giuseppe, M.D., Maria Maglio, M.D., Carlo Cuni, M.D., et al. "Poor

Glucose Control in the Year before Admission as a Powerful Predictor of Amputation in Hospitalized Patients with Foot Ulceration." *Diabetes Care* (August 2006) 29: 1985.

Lyssenko, Valeriya, M.D., et al. "Clinical Risk Factors, DNA Variants, and the Development of Type 2 Diabetes." *New England Journal of Medicine* (20 November 2008) 359: 2220–2232.

Margolis, David J., M.D., Ole Hofstad, and Harold I. Feldman, M.D. "The Association between Renal Failure and Foot Ulcer or Lower Extremity Amputation in Patients with Diabetes." *Diabetes Care* (July 2008) 31: 1331–1336.

McClain, Carla. "Southern Arizona, Epicenter of an Epidemic." (Tucson) *Arizona Daily Star*, 18 July 2004.

McEwen, Laura M., William H. Herman, M.D., et al. "Diabetes Reporting as a Cause of Death, Results from the Translating Results into Action for Diabetes (TRIAD) Study." *Diabetes Care* (February 2006) 29: 247–253.

Meigs, James B., M.D., et al. "Genotype Score in Addition to Common Risk Factors for Prediction of Type 2 Diabetes." *New England Journal of Medicine* (20 November 2008) 359: 2208–2219.

Meyer-Davis, Elizabeth J., et al. "Breast-Feeding and Risk for Childhood Obesity." *Diabetes Care* (October 2006) 29: 2231–2237.

Moses, Robert G., M.D., Megan Barker, A.P.D., Meagen Winter, A.P.D., Peter Petocz, Ph.D., Jennie C. Brand-Miller, Ph.D. "Can a Low-Glycemic Index Diet Reduce the Need for Insulin in Gestational Diabetes Mellitus?" *Diabetes Care* (June 19, 2009) 32: 996–1000.

Munshi, Medha, M.D., et al. "Cognitive Dysfunction Is Associated with Poor Diabetes Control in Older Adults." *Diabetes Care* (August 2006) 29: 1794–1700.

Mutch, David M., and Karine Clement. "Unraveling the Genetics of Human Obesity." PLoS Genetics. (29 December 2006) 2 (12): e 188.

Mulvaney, Shelagh A., et al. "Parent Perceptions for Adolescents with Type 2 Diabetes." *Diabetes Care* (May 2006) 29: 993–997.

Murphy, Sean. "Oklahoma City Mayor Puts City on a Diet." Associated Press,

3 January 2008; archived at www.msnbc.msn.com/id/22503467/.

Narayan, K.M. Venkat, et al. "Impact of Recent Increase on Future Diabetes Burden, U.S. 2005–2050." *Diabetes Care* (September 2006) 29: 2114–6.

Nathan, David M., MD (Chair), The International Expert Committee, International Expert Committee Report on the Role of the A1C Assay in the Diagnoses of Diabetes, *Diabetes Care* 32: 1327–1334, July 2009.

Neil, H., W. Andrew, et al. "Collaborative Atrovastatin Diabetes Study (CARDS), Analysis of Efficacy and Safety in Patients Aged 65–75 Years at Randomization." *Diabetes Care* (November 2006) 29: 2378–2384.

Nilsson, Peter, M.D., and Leif Groop, M.D. "Clinical Risk Factors, DNA Variants, and the Development of Type 2 Diabetes." *New England Journal of Medicine* (20 November 2008) 359: 2220–2232.

Oomichi, Takeisi, M.D., Masonori Emoto, M.D., et al. "Impact of Glycemic Control on Survival of Diabetic Patients on Chronic Regular Hemodialysis, a 7-year Observational Study." *Diabetes Care* (July 2006) 29: 1496–1500.

Perez-Pena, Richard. "As Increase in Diabetes Destroys More Kidneys, New York Dialysis Lags." *The New York Times*, 28 December 2006.

Phelan, Suzanne, Alka M. Kanaya, M.D., Leslee L. Subak, M.D., et al. "Prevalence and Risk Factors for Urinary Incontinence in Overweight and Obese Diabetic Women." *Diabetes Care* (August 2009) 32: 1391–1397.

Philbrick, Nathaniel. *In the Heart of the Sea: The Tragedy of the Whaleship Essex*. New York: Penguin, 2000.

Pollack, Andrew. "The Dialysis Business: Fair Treatment?" *The New York Times*, 16 September 2007.

Racette, Susan B., Ellen M. Evans, Edward P. Weiss, et al. "Abdominal Adiposity Is a Stronger Predictor of Insulin Resistance than Fitness among 50 to 95 Year Olds." *Diabetes Care* (2006) 29: 673–678.

Ratner, Robert, M.D. "Prevention of Type 2 Diabetes in Women with Previous Gestational Diabetes." *Diabetes Care* (July 2007, supplement 2) 30: s242–s245.

Ratsimamanga, Urverg Suzanne. "Eugenia Jambolana: Madagascar." Malagasy Institute of Applied Research. Retrieved from http://tcdc.undp.org/SIE/experiences/vol7/Eugenia%20Jambolana_Madagascar.pdf.

Reader, Diane M. "Medical Nutrition Therapy and Life Style Interventions." *Diabetes Care* (July 2007, supplement 2) 30: s188–s193.

Resnick, Helane E., Janice Heineman, Robin Stone, et al. "Diabetes in U.S. Nursing Homes, 2004." *Diabetes Care* (February 2008) 31: 287–288.

Rubino, Francesco, M.D. "Is Type 2 Diabetes an Operable Intestinal Disease? A Provocative yet Reasonable Hypothesis." *Diabetes Care* (February 2008, supplement 2) 31: s290–s296.

Ryan, Christopher M., et al. "Improving Metabolic Control Leads to Better Working Memory in Adults with Type 2 Diabetes." *Diabetes Care* (February 2006) 20: 345–351.

Ryan, Marie E., Oana Carnu, and Ruth Tenzler. "The Impact of Periodontitis on Metabolic Control and Risk for Diabetic Complications." *RDH Magazine*, 19 July 2007, archived at www.rdhmag.com/display_article/300572/108/none/none/Oart/THE-IMPACT-OF-PERIODONTITIS-ON-METABOLIC-CONTROL-AND-RISK-FOR-DIABETIC-COMPLICTION.

Sam, Susan, M.D., Steven Haffner, M.D., Michael A. Davidson, M.D., Ralph B. Dagostino, Sr., M.D., Steven Feinstein, M.D., George Kondos, M.D., Alphonso Perez, M.D., Theodore Mazzone, M.D. "Relation of Abdominal Fat Deposits to Systemic Markers of Inflammation in Type 2 Diabetes." *Diabetes Care* (May 2009) 32: 932–937.

Sardinha, Louis B., et al. "Objectively Measured Time Spent Sedentary Is Associated with Insulin Resistance Independent of Overall and Central Body Fat in 9- to 10-Year-Old Portuguese Children." *Diabetes Care* (March 2008) 31: 569–575.

Schernithaner, Guntram, M.D., and John M. Morton, M.D. "Bariatric Surgery in Patients with Morbid Obesity and Type 2 Diabetes." *Diabetes Care* (February 2008 supplement 2) 30: s297–s302.

Schofield, Christopher J., Andrew D. Morris, M.D., et al. "Mortality and Hospitalization in Patients after Amputation, a Comparison between Patients with and without Diabetes." *Diabetes Care* (2006) 29: 2252–2256.

Schulz, Leslie O., Peter H. Bennett, et al. "Effects of Traditional and Western Environments on Prevalence of Type 2 Diabetes in Pima Indians in Mexico and the U.S." *Diabetes Care* (August 2006) 29: 1866–1871.

Selven, Elizabeth, Josef Coresh, M.D., and Frederick L. Brancati, M.D. "The Burden and Treatment of Diabetes in Elderly Individuals in the U.S." *Diabetes Care* (November 2006) 29: 2415–2419.

Shah, Pankaj, Jeffrey Cui, Naifa L. Busaidy, Steven I. Sherman, and Victor R. Lavis. "Why is 'New' Hyperglycemia Dangerous in the Cancer Hospital?" (Abstract #1033-P). Lecture presented at the American Diabetes Scientific Sessions, San Francisco, June 2008. Online at American Diabetes Association website; Diabetes PRO.

Shai, Iris, Rui Jiang, M.D., et al. "Ethnicity, Obesity, and Risk of Type 2 Diabetes in Women, a Twenty Year Follow-Up Study." *Diabetes Care* (July 2006) 29: 1585–1590.

Shaw, Milissa, Mary Savoye, Anna Calle, M.D., et al. "Effect of a Successful Lifestyle Program on Insulin Sensitivity and Glucose Tolerance in Obese Youth." *Diabetes Care* (January 2009) 32: 45–47.

Shepherd, V.A. "Bioelectricity and the Rhythms of Sensitive Plants: The Biophysical Research of Jagadis Chandra Bose." *Current Science Online*. www.ias.ac.in/currsci/jul10/articles33.htm.

Ship, Jonathan A. "Diabetes and Oral Health: An Overview." *Journal of the American Dental Association* (4 April 2003) 134: 4S–10S.

Skutch, Andrew. *The Life of the Hummingbird*. New York: Vintage Books, 1973.

Skyler, Jay S., M.D., et al. "Intensive Glycemic Control and the Prevention of Cardiovascular Events: Implications of the ACCORD, ADVANCE, and VA Diabetes Trials." *Diabetes Care* (2009) 32:187–192.

Smith, A. Gordon, M.D., et al. "Life Style Intervention for Pre-Diabetic Neuropathy." *Diabetes Care* (June 2006) 29: 1204–1299.

Sorensen, Lea, Linda Molyneaux, and Dennis K. Yue. "The Relationship among Pain, Sensory Loss, and Small Nerve Fibers in Diabetes." *Diabetes Care* (April 2006) 29: 883–887.

Stratton, I.M., et al. "Association of Glycemia with Macrovascular and Microvascular Complications of Type 2 Diabetes (UKPDS 35): Prospective Observational Study." *British Medical Journal* (2000) 321: 405–412.

Thorpe, Lorna E., et al. "Prevalence and Control of Diabetes and Impaired Fasting Glucose in New York City." *Diabetes Care* (January 2009) 32: 57–62.

Tonetti, Maurizio S., et al. "Treatment of Periodontitis and Endothelial Function." *The New England Journal of Medicine* (1 March 2007) 356: 911–920.

Tuomi, Thnamaija, M.D., Elena H. Honkanen, M.D., et al. "Improved Prandial Glucose Control with Lower Risk of Hypoglycemia with Nateglinide than with Glibenclamide in Patients with Maturity-Onset Diabetes of the Young Type 3." *Diabetes Care* (February 2006) 29:189–194.

Tuomilehto, J., et al. "Effects of Calcium-Channel Blockade in Older Patients with Diabetes and Systolic Hypertension." *New England Journal of Medicine* (1999) 340: 677–684.

Tushuizen, Maarten E., M.D., Mathis C. Bunk, M.D., et al. "Pancreatic Fat Content and B-Cell Function in Men with and without Type 2 Diabetes." *Diabetes Care* (November 2007) 30: 2916–2921.

Unger, Roger H. "Weapons of Lean Body Mass Destruction: The Role of Lipids in the Metabolic Syndrome." *Endocrinology* (2003) 144: 5159–5165.

Unger, Roger H., Yan Tang Zhou, and Lelio Orci. "Regulation of Fatty Acid Homeostasis in Cells: Novel Role of Leptin." *Proceedings of the National Academy of Sciences* (2 March 1999) 96(5): 2327–2332.

Wackers, Frans J. Th., M.D., et al. "Resolution of Asymptomatic Myocardial Ischemia in Patients with Type 2 Diabetes in the Detection of Ischemia in Asymptomatic Diabetics (DIAD) Study." *Diabetes Care* (November 2007) 30: 2892–2898.

Wind, Debra Siefried. "Type 2 Diabetes, Obesity and Bumblefoot: A Possible Correlation?" *Rat and Mouse Gazette*, June 2003, archived at www.rmca.org/Articles/diabetestype2.htm.

Xue, Jay L., Jennie Z. Ma, Thomas A. Lewis, and Allan J. Collins. "Forecast of the Number of Dialysis Patients in the United States to the Year 2010." *Journal of the American Society of Nephrology* (2001) 12: 2753–2758.

Yaggi, H. Klar, M.D., Ansdre B. Araujo, and John B. McKinley. "Sleep Deprivation as a Risk Factor for Type 2 Diabetes." *Diabetes Care* (March 2006) 29: 657–661.

Yokoyama, H., M. Okudaria, A. Sato, et al. "Higher Incidence of Diabetic Neuropathy in Type 2 than in Type1 Diabetics in Early Onset Diabetes in Japan." *Kidney International* (2000) 58: 302–311.

Zhang, Cuilin, M.D., Simin Liu, M.D., Caren G. Solomon, M.D., and Frank B. Hu, M.D. "Dietary Fiber Intake, Dietary Glycemic Load, and the Risk for Diabetes Mellitus." *Diabetes Care* (October 2006) 29: 2223–2230.

Other Internet Sources

The problem of unexploded land mines: http://www.unicef.org/graca/mines.htm.

Maturity onset diabetes of the young:
- At diabetesgenes.org: projects.exeter.ac.uk/diabetesgenes/mody/index.
- At Wikipedia: http://en.wikipedia.org/wiki/Maturity_onset_diabetes_in_the_young

Samuel Rahbar and origin of HbA1c: http://en.wikipedia.org/wiki/Samuel_Rahbar

History of hemodialysis: http://www.fmc-ag.com/internet/fmc/fmcag/neu/fmcpub.nsf/Content/Dialysis_Compact_2004_0.

Diabetes data and trends from the U.S. Centers for Disease Control and Prevention: http://apps.nccd.cdc.gov/ddtstrs/.

INDEX

Numbers in *bold italics* indicate pages with illustrations.

225

tax burden of diabetes 209
team approach to diabetes care 152
Tenkoff peritoneal dialysis catheter 173
Thrifty Gene Theory 49, 50
thrombolytic agents 159
Thurber, James 98
Tohono O'odham Indians 46–49
transient ischemic attack (TIA) 176, 184,
    194; *see also* ministroke
triglycerides 61, 95, 96
trophic ulceration 99, *100*
Tucker, Ellen 7
Type 3c Diabetes 31, 32

universal health care 138
University of Medicine and Dentistry of
    New Jersey 6
University of Michigan 49
University of Tehran 37
urinary incontinence 91
urinary retention 91

vagal reaction 176
vas deferens calcification 205

vegetarian 94
visceral fat 56
visual impairment 195

Waddington, Conrad Hal 48
waist circumference 25, 56
water tasters 24
Watson, James 48
weight reduction surgery *see* metabolic
    surgery
whirlpool treatment 91, 122
Whitney, Eli 53
World Health Organization 9, 171
wound care centers 122
wound dressing technique (wet-to-damp)
    123, *124*, 125
wound healing 117–120

xerostomia (dry eye) 100, 198

Yale University 45, 208

Zucker, Lois 59–61
Zucker, Dr. Theodore 59–61